-Nurturing Wellness-
THE PATH TO POSTMENOPAUSAL HEART DISEASE AWARENESS

Empowering Women to Understand Menopause and Heart Health, Taking Control for a Vibrant Life Beyond Menopause

DR. DINESH KANFADE

Disclaimer:

While the publisher and author have used their best efforts in preparing this book, they make no representation or warranties with respect to the accuracy or completeness of the contents of this book and specifically disclaim any implied warranties of merchantability or fitness for a particular purpose. No warranty may be created or extended by sales representatives or written sales materials. The advice and strategies contained herein may not be suitable for your situation. This book is for educational purpose only. It is not intended for the substitute for the diagnosis, treatment and advice of a qualified licensed professional. You should consult your healthcare provider for individualized advice. Neither the publisher nor the author shall be liable for any other commercial damages, including but not limited to special, incidental, consequential, personal, or other damage.

ACKNOWLEDGEMENTS

I wish to express my gratitude to various sources, knowingly or unknowingly has contributed for empowering my knowledge, empowering women's health and helping me to write this book.

I would like to thank my mentors and teachers who had been a torch bearer for me for writing this book.

I am extremely thankful to **Dr. Suresh Sonawane** Sr. Consultant Physician for taking time from his busy schedule to write **"FOREWORD"** for my book.

I am also thankful to **Dr. Anamika Samant** Sr. Consultant Physician for taking time from her busy schedule to write **"FOREWORD"** for my book.

Book images Credit and Courtesy: *

The Heart and Large Vessels: **Henry Vandyke / Henry Gray / Wikimedia Commons**

Blood Oxygenation to the Pulmonary and Systemic Circulation: **Sasha River Santilla / Wikimedia Commons**

Illustration of Atherosclerotic Changes: **Freepik.com**

I also express my sincere gratitude to my family members and friends who have always been supportive and motivated me in my initiatives in writing series of books on **"Women's Health"**, this book being eighth in the series.

DEDICATION

Dedicated to my better half Nita, son Akshay, daughter-in-law Priya and little sweet Avni.

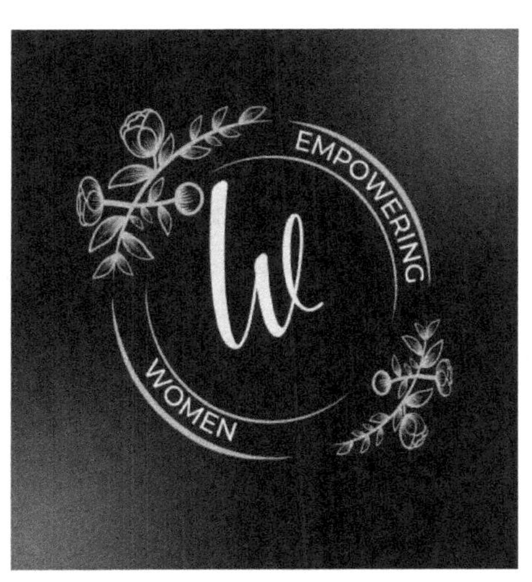

EMPOWERING
WOMEN

"Low Carbohydrate, High Protein Diet and Muscle Strengthening can Decrease fat, Lead to Good Body Shape, can Reverse Diabetes, Decrease Pains, Decrease Heart Attacks, Lead to Stronger Bones, Reduce Your Doctor Visits and can Have a Vibrant Life Beyond Menopause."

FOREWORD

I am delighted to write a foreword for the book, **"Nurturing Wellness: The Path to Postmenopausal Heart Disease Awareness"** authored by Dr. Dinesh Kanfade.

As we advance in medical science, it has become clear that women health, particularly during and after menopause, deserve special attention. In the book titled, **"Nurturing Wellness: The Path to Postmenopausal Heart Disease Awareness"**, the author sheds light on a critical, often overlooked connection between menopause and cardiovascular disease. This book is not only informative but also empowering, guiding women through the unique challenges they face in protecting their heart health during this stage of life.

By addressing both misconceptions and specific risk factors, the author equips readers with practical tools to take control of their health. This timely and well-researched work will undoubtedly become a vital resource for women, healthcare professionals and anyone dedicated to improve women's heart health.

DR. SURESH SONAWANE

MD (Internal Medicine) Mumbai University

Sr. Consultant Physician

Medical Director, Sankalp Hospital & ICCU,

Virar-West-401303.

FOREWORD

It is my privilege to present the book, **"Nurturing Wellness: The Path to Postmenopausal Heart Disease Awareness"** written by Dr. Dinesh Kanfade.

This comprehensive guide delves into the women's cardiovascular health, offering clarity on misconceptions, traditional and women-specific risk factors, and the profound impact of menopause on heart health. The author skillfully bridges the gap between medical insights and practical advice, empowering readers to take charge of their well-being. This book doesn't inform, but it urges women to embrace lifestyle modifications that can significantly reduce the risk of cardiovascular disease.

Cardiovascular disease is the number one killer in postmenopausal women, cancer being second. Heart health often takes a backseat in women's lives, especially during postmenopausal years when other priorities seem to be more pressing. However, this stage brings unique challenges that demand urgent attention and awareness. I am confident that this book will stand as a beacon of hope and a resource for both healthcare professionals and the women navigating their postmenopausal years.

DR. ANAMIKA SAMANT

DNB (Internal Medicine), PGD Obesity Management (USW, Cardiff), FICP, FDI.

Sr. Consultant Physician

Chaitanya Hospital & Obesity Clinic, Virar.

PREFACE

"To keep the body in good health is a duty…otherwise we shall not be able to keep our mind strong"
-Buddha

The biggest achievement of the last century is greater longevity that has resulted in increasing aged population worldwide. It is obvious that women have to live significant part of their lives after menopause. Menopause transition bring profound hormonal changes that can affect multiple aspects of health, including an often-overlooked issue: cardiovascular disease (CVD). Heart disease is the leading cause of death among women in postmenopausal age group, cancer being second. Yet many women are unaware of the heightened risk of CVD they face after menopause. The benefit of increased lifespan is only when it is translated into healthy aging.

This book, **"Nurturing Wellness: The Path to Postmenopausal Heart Disease Awareness"**, highlights the importance of understanding cardiovascular health during this crucial phase of life. In addition to the risk factors common to both genders, women experience unique risk factors such as the decline in estrogen level during menopause transition, which increases vulnerability to heart disease. Furthermore, complications from pregnancy, such as preeclampsia, gestational diabetes, bad obstetric history or preterm delivery, add to the complexity of CVD risks in later years. Traditional heart disease symptoms may also present differently in women, making awareness even more essential.

To help women take charge of their heart health, this book provides actionable lifestyle strategies, including dietary supplements, exercise routines, stress management and the importance of regular screening. The goal is to empower women with knowledge and tools to prevent and manage cardiovascular disease proactively.

Through a blend of science, practical advice and personal empowerment, this book serves as a comprehensive guide for women, healthcare professionals and caregivers. Let's embrace this conversation about menopause and cardiovascular health – because awareness and the action today can lead to healthier and happier lives tomorrow.

"With healthy lifestyle and better understanding of cardiovascular health during menopause transition, not only years will be added to increase the lifespan, but the extra years added will be of good quality."

DR. DINESH KANFADE

MBBS, DGO, DFP, FICMCH, CIMP.

Sr. Obstetrician & Gynecologist

Table of Contents

CHAPTER I: INTRODUCTION

"Postmenopausal women face a unique set of cardiovascular challenges; understanding these challenges is key to having heart-healthy life."

(A)Why Risk for Cardiovascular Disease is to be Taken Seriously in Postmenopausal Women?

Cardiovascular disease (CVD) in postmenopausal women is a serious concern due to several physiological and hormonal changes that increase the risk of heart disease. Here are some key points highlighting this importance:

1. **Increased Risk of Cardiovascular Disease (CVD):**
   After menopause, women experience a sharp decline in estrogen levels, a hormone that has a protective effect on the heart and blood vessels.

2. **Changes in Cholesterol Levels:**
   Postmenopausal women often see a rise in LDL (bad cholesterol) and a decrease in HDL (good cholesterol) levels, which can contribute to the buildup of plaque in the arteries, increasing the risk of atherosclerosis.

3. **Blood Pressure:**
   Menopause is associated with an increase in blood pressure. The loss of estrogen can make blood vessels less flexible, leading to higher blood pressure, which is a significant risk factor for heart disease.

4. **Weight Gain and Metabolic Changes:**
   Many women gain weight during menopause, particularly the visceral fat, which can increase the risk of metabolic syndrome – a group of conditions that elevate the risk of heart disease, stroke and diabetes.

5. **Diabetes Mellitus:**
   The risk of developing type 2 diabetes increases after menopause, partly due to weight gain and changes in body fat distribution. Diabetes is a major risk factor for diabetes.

6. **Inflammation:**
   Menopause is associated with increased levels of inflammation in the body, which can contribute to the development of atherosclerosis and other cardiovascular conditions.

7. **Lifestyle Factors:**
   The transition into menopause often coincides with lifestyle changes, such as reduced physical activity, poor diet, and increased stress, all of which can further elevate cardiovascular risk.

Addressing cardiovascular health in postmenopausal women is essential for early intervention so as to improve their overall quality of life and reducing the risk of serious life-threatening conditions.

(B)Greater Longevity:

Increased longevity for women is a significant global and regional trend, reflecting improvements in healthcare, living conditions, and overall quality of life. Here's a look at how women's life expectancy has changed globally and in India over time:

Global Trends

Historical Perspective:

- **Early 20th Century**: In the early 1900s, global life expectancy for women was significantly lower, often below 50 years in many regions. High mortality rates from infectious diseases, poor maternal health, and limited medical advancements contributed to this lower life expectancy.

- **Mid to Late 20th Century**: Improvements in healthcare, vaccination programs, better nutrition, and advancements in medical technology led to a gradual increase in life expectancy. By the end of the 20th century, women's life expectancy had risen substantially, reaching an average of about 72 years globally.

Current Data:

- **Global Life Expectancy**: As of recent data, the global life expectancy for women is around 75 years. This figure reflects continued advancements in healthcare, reduced child mortality, and improved management of chronic diseases.

- **Regional Variations**: Life expectancy varies significantly by region, with higher figures in developed countries (often exceeding 80 years) and lower figures in developing regions.

Trends in India

Historical Perspective:

- **Pre-Independence Era**: Life expectancy in India was quite low before the mid-20th century, with women often living to around 30-40 years due to high infant mortality rates, maternal health issues, and limited healthcare infrastructure.

- **Post-Independence Improvements**: Since independence in 1947, India has seen significant improvements in healthcare, sanitation, and nutrition, contributing to increased life expectancy.

Current Data:

- **Life Expectancy**: As of recent estimates, the life expectancy for women in India is approximately 73 years. This is a marked improvement from previous decades and reflects progress in health care, disease control, and living conditions.

- **Regional Disparities**: Life expectancy varies within India, with higher figures in urban areas compared to rural regions. States with better healthcare infrastructure and socioeconomic conditions tend to have higher life expectancies.

Factors Contributing to Increased Longevity:

- **Healthcare Advancements**: Improvements in medical care, including access to vaccines, better management of chronic diseases, and advanced treatments, have significantly contributed to longer lifespans.

- **Nutritional Improvements**: Enhanced access to a varied and nutritious diet has led to better overall health and increased longevity.

- **Sanitation and Public Health**: Improvements in sanitation, clean drinking water, and public health measures have reduced mortality rates from infectious diseases and improved quality of life.

- **Education and Awareness**: Greater awareness about health, preventive measures, and lifestyle changes has played a role in increasing life expectancy.

- **Economic Development**: Economic growth has led to improved living standards, better healthcare access, and increased longevity.

Challenges and Considerations:

- **Chronic Diseases**: While longevity has increased, there is a growing burden of chronic diseases such as cardiovascular diseases, diabetes, and cancer, which are more prevalent in older age.

- **Healthcare Access**: In both global and Indian contexts, disparities in healthcare access can impact longevity and quality of life, particularly in underserved regions.

The increased longevity of women globally and in India reflects significant progress in health and living conditions. However, this extended lifespan also brings challenges related to managing chronic diseases and ensuring equitable access to healthcare. Ongoing efforts in healthcare improvement, public health, and socioeconomic development are essential to addressing these challenges and improving the quality of life for older women.

While longevity has contributed to an increase in cardiovascular disease cases due to the aging population, medical advancements, lifestyle interventions, and early detection have made it possible to manage these conditions effectively. Thus, while increased life expectancy had led to a greater prevalence of CVD, it has also provided opportunities to better understand, prevent and treat these diseases, ultimately promoting healthier aging and longer lives. Benefit of increased longevity is only when it is translated into healthy aging.

(C)Statistics on Cardiovascular Disease in Postmenopausal Women

Global Statistics:

Cardiovascular disease (CVD) is the leading cause of death among postmenopausal women worldwide, with significant gender-specific risk factors emerging after menopause. Here are some key global statistics:

1. **Prevalence of CVD in Women:**
    *   According to the **World Health Organization (WHO),** approximately 17.9 million people die from CVD each year, with nearly 7.4 million women affected globally.

    *   After menopause the cardiovascular diseases, including coronary artery disease and stroke, increases by 2 – 3 times due to the decline in estrogen levels.

    *   Heart disease account for nearly one-third of all deaths in women globally, surpassing even cancer as the leading cause of death.

2. **Age and CVD risk in Postmenopausal Women:**
    *   The risk of coronary heart disease (CHD) increases markedly after age 50, corelating with the onset of menopause. Women aged 55 and above face a significant higher risk of developing heart disease.

    *   A report from American Heart Association (AHA) found that approximately one in three women will suffer from cardiovascular disease after

menopause, with around 70% of heart attacks in women occurring after the age of 55.

3. **Deaths from CVD:**
   - Globally, CVD causes over 8.6 million deaths among women each year, making up 35% of all female deaths worldwide.

   - Postmenopausal women have a 50% higher chance of dying from heart disease compared to premenopausal women.

Indian Scenario:

India faces a growing burden of cardiovascular disease, and postmenopausal women are among the most vulnerable groups due to gender-specific risk factors. Here are some notable statistics:

1. **Increasing Prevalence in Women:**
   - A study from the Indian Heart Association highlights that postmenopausal women in India are at increasing risk, with CVD prevalence at around 18 – 20% in women aged 55 and older.

   - In India, 52% of women over 50 have some form of heart disease, with this figure rising among postmenopausal women due to factors like diabetes, hypertension, and sedentary lifestyle.

2. **Mortality from Cardiovascular Disease:**
   - Cardiovascular diseases are responsible for about 25% of all female deaths in India.

- Women in India have a higher rate of premature cardiovascular deaths compared to the global average, with one in four women succumbing to heart disease before reaching 70.

3. **Risk Factors in Postmenopausal Women:**
   - The incidence of hypertension in postmenopausal women in India is around 30 – 35%, one of the leading contributors to cardiovascular disease.

   - Diabetes prevalence is significantly higher in postmenopausal women, contributing to their increased risk of heart disease. Nearly 25% of postmenopausal women in urban India have diabetes, while in rural areas, this figure stands at around 15 – 20%.

4. **Health Disparities:**
   - Studies have shown that postmenopausal women from lower socioeconomic groups, particularly in rural India, face a higher burden of CVD, with less access to healthcare and preventive measures.

   - A 2019 report found that 72% of postmenopausal women in India have never been screened for heart disease, highlighting significant gaps in awareness and healthcare access.

These statistics emphasize the growing impact of cardiovascular disease on postmenopausal women, globally and in India. Given the unique risk factors faced by women after menopause, focused prevention and education efforts are crucial to reduce the burden of cardiovascular disease in this population.

As per the CDC Report (Centre for Disease Control and Prevention):

- Despite an increase in awareness over the past decades, only about half (56%) of women recognize that heart disease is their number one killer, cancer being second.

- Heart is the leading cause of death for women in United States, killing 314186 women in 2020: or about 1 in every 5 female deaths.

- Although heart disease was initially thought of as a man's disease, almost as many women as men die of heart disease each year in menopausal age group in United States.

(D)Misconceptions About Cardiovascular Health in Postmenopausal Women:

Here are some misconceptions about postmenopausal cardiovascular health, followed by the facts that address them:

1. **Misconception:**
    Cardiovascular disease is a man's health issue.

    Fact: Cardiovascular disease is the leading cause of death in women, particularly after menopause. The drop in estrogen levels post-menopause significantly increases a woman's risk for heart disease.

2. **Misconception:**
    Only women with obvious risk factors (e.g., high blood pressure, smoking) need to worry about heart health after menopause.

    Fact: All women are at risk of cardiovascular disease after menopause, even those with traditional risk factors. Declining estrogen, obesity, and other metabolic changes contribute to this risk.

3. **Misconception:**
    Weight gain after menopause is inevitable and not related to heart heath.

    Fact: While weight gain can be common after menopause, it has significant implications for heart health. Increased abdominal (visceral) fat contributes to a higher risk of heart disease and metabolic disorders like diabetes.

4. **Misconception:**
    Postmenopausal women need not bother about cholesterol levels if premenopausal cholesterol levels were normal all the time.

    Fact: Menopause often leads to unfavorable changes in cholesterol levels, including increased LDL (bad cholesterol) and decreased HDL (good cholesterol), which can elevate the risk for heart disease, even if premenopausal cholesterol levels were normal all the time.

5. **Misconception:**
    Cardiovascular symptoms in women are the same as in men.

    Fact: Women often experience different and more subtle symptoms of heart disease, such as fatigue, nausea, and back pain, which can be mistaken for other conditions. They are less likely to have classical retrosternal chest pain like men and hence sometimes diagnosis can be missed.

6. **Misconception:**
    Physical activity doesn't make a difference after menopause.

    Fact: Regular physical activity is crucial in reducing the risk of cardiovascular disease in postmenopausal women. It helps manage weight, improve heart function, and control blood pressure and cholesterol levels.

7. **Misconception:**
Heart disease won't be a concern as long as blood pressure is under control.

Fact: While keeping blood pressure under control is important, other factors like cholesterol levels, glucose levels, inflammation, and lifestyle choices (diet, exercise) also significantly impact heart health.

8. **Misconception:**
Once a woman reaches menopause, there is nothing she can do to lower the risk of heart disease.

Fact: Postmenopausal women can still reduce their chances of getting heart disease by adopting healthy lifestyle, including maintaining a heart-friendly balanced diet, engaging in regular exercise, managing stress, and monitoring their heart health regularly.

9. **Misconception:**
Menopause-related symptoms like hot flashes and night sweats may not have an increased risk of cardiovascular disease.

Fact: Some studies suggest that women who experience frequent or severe hot flashes and night sweats may have an increased risk of cardiovascular disease, indicating that these symptoms could be early markers for heart disease.

10. **Misconception:**
Hormone Replacement Therapy (HRT) protects heart disease and can be stared at any time postmenopause.

Fact: According to the recommendations of HRT, it is not recommended for primary or secondary prevention of cardiovascular disease. But if started for another indication like hot flashes and night sweats within 6 years of postmenopause, it can prove beneficial for heart health.

These misconceptions highlight the importance of awareness and proactive heart health management for postmenopausal women.

(E)Objective of Writing a Book

The objective of writing a book titled, **"Nurturing Wellness: The Path to Postmenopausal Heart Disease Awareness"** would be multifaceted, aiming to address critical and often overlooked under-represented connection between menopause and cardiovascular health.

The primary objectives include:

- **Raising Awareness:**
  To educate women, healthcare professionals, and the general public about the increased risk of cardiovascular disease (CVD) in postmenopausal women, which is the leading cause of mortality but often overlooked in discussions about women's health.

- **Providing Evidence-Based Information:**
  To present the latest research, statistics, and clinical evidence on how menopause and the associated decline in estrogen levels impact cardiovascular health. This would include information on risk factors, symptoms, and physiological changes that contribute to increased cardiovascular health.

- **Empowering Women:**
  To empower postmenopausal women with knowledge about their cardiovascular health so they can make informed decisions about life choices, preventive measures, and treatment options. The book would aim to guide women in understanding their unique health needs during this stage of life.

- **Offering Practical Advice:**
  To provide practical strategies for maintaining and improving cardiovascular health post-menopause. This

might include lifestyle modifications such as diet, exercise, stress management, and the role of hormone replacement therapy (HRT) and other medical interventions.

- **Heightened Gender-specific Research and Care:**
  To emphasize the importance of gender-specific research and the need for healthcare systems to recognize and address the unique cardiovascular risks faced by postmenopausal women. The book could advocate for more tailored healthcare approaches and support for women.

- **Promoting Early Detection and Prevention:**
  To encourage early detection and prevention of cardiovascular diseases in postmenopausal women through regular screenings, monitoring of risk factors, and proactive health management. The book would stress the importance of routine check-ups and communication with healthcare providers.

- **Addressing Common Myths and Misconceptions:**
  To debunk common myths and misconceptions about menopause and cardiovascular health.

- **Supporting Holistic Health:**
  To promote a holistic approach to postmenopausal health, considering the interplay between cardiovascular health and other aspects of physical, mental and emotional well-being. The book could explore how factors like stress, mental health, and overall lifestyle influence cardiovascular health.

- **Advocating for Policy and Social Change:**
  To advocate for greater attention to women's health policy, especially focusing on cardiovascular disease prevention for postmenopausal women.

By addressing these objectives, the book would serve as a comprehensive resource that fills a critical gap in both academic and practical health guidance for postmenopausal women, ultimately contributing to quality of life.

Target Audience:

- **Postmenopausal Women**: Primary audience seeking information on how to manage their cardiovascular health.

- **Healthcare Providers**: Gynecologists, and primary care physicians looking for a resource to better support their postmenopausal patients.

- **Caregivers and Family Members**: Individuals supporting postmenopausal women who want to understand cardiovascular health.

- **General Readers**: Anyone interested in learning more about the intersection of menopause and cardiovascular health.

(F)Inspiring Story of a Vibrant Woman

The Wake-Up Call

Nita was a vibrant 59-year-old woman living in a small, picturesque town nestled in the rolling hills of India. A retired high school teacher, Nita spent her days gardening, volunteering at the local library, and enjoying time with her grandchildren. Life was good, but something had changed recently. She noticed she was feeling unusually fatigued, often had shortness of breath, and her doctor had warned her that her cholesterol levels were rising. Nita was postmenopausal, and her annual check-up revealed that she was at an increased risk of cardiovascular disease.

The diagnosis was a jolt to Nita. Her mother had passed away from heart disease at a relatively young age, and Nita had always feared she might face the same fate. Determined to change her path, she set out to learn more about managing her health.

The Quest for Knowledge

Nita began her journey by attending a community health seminar organized by a local hospital. The seminar featured a cardiologist, a dietitian, and a fitness trainer. The cardiologist explained the connection between menopause and cardiovascular risk, emphasizing the importance of diet and exercise. The dietitian discussed the benefits of a heart-healthy diet, rich in fruits, vegetables, whole grains, and lean proteins, while the fitness trainer highlighted the role of regular physical activity in maintaining cardiovascular health.

Nita soaked up the information like a sponge. She learned about the Mediterranean diet, which was high in healthy fats from sources like olive oil and nuts, and how reducing processed foods and excess salt could improve her heart health. She also discovered the importance of regular exercise, not just for weight management but for overall heart health.

A New Beginning

Empowered by her newfound knowledge, Nita made significant changes to her lifestyle. She started by overhauling her diet, incorporating more fresh produce and whole grains into her meals. She also began a daily exercise routine, including brisk walking and strength training, which she found invigorating and enjoyable. Her efforts paid off. Over the next few months, Nita's cholesterol levels improved, her energy returned, and she felt more confident about her health. The changes in her lifestyle not only benefited her physically but also mentally, as she felt more in control of her well-being.

Becoming an Advocate

Inspired by her own transformation, Nita decided to help others in her community. She started volunteering with the local health department, organizing workshops and seminars on heart disease prevention. Her personal story resonated with many, and she became a passionate advocate for cardiovascular health.

Nita also began writing a blog where she shared tips on healthy eating, exercise routines, and the emotional aspects of managing health. Her blog quickly gained a following, and she was invited to speak at local events and health fairs.

She partnered with healthcare professionals to create a community support group for women at risk of cardiovascular disease. The group provided education, encouragement, and a platform for sharing experiences. Nita's initiative led to regular meetings where participants could learn from experts and support each other in making healthier choices.

The Ripple Effect

Nita's efforts had a profound impact on her community. Many women who attended her workshops and read her blogs reported improvements in their health and well-being. Local health metrics showed a decrease in cardiovascular risk factors among the participants, and the community began to embrace healthier lifestyles more broadly.

Nita's journey from a concerned patient to a community advocate highlighted the power of knowledge and the importance of proactive health management. Her story became an inspiring example of how individuals can turn personal challenges into opportunities to make a difference in the lives of others.

As she looked back on her journey, Nita felt a deep sense of fulfillment. Her efforts had not only improved her own health but had also empowered many others to take charge of their cardiovascular health. She knew that her work was far from over, but she was confident that with continued education and support, more lives would be transformed for the better.

And so, Nita continued her advocacy, her heart full of hope and determination, knowing that every small step toward a healthier lifestyle could make a big difference in preventing cardiovascular disease and fostering a healthier, more informed community.

CHAPTER II: UNDERSTANDING CARDIOVASCULAR SYSTEM

"Knowledge is the first step towards empowerment;

understanding basic anatomy and physiology

is vital for women's health journey"

(A)Basic Cardiovascular Anatomy and Physiology

The cardiovascular system, also known as the circulatory system, is responsible for the transportation of blood, nutrients, oxygen, carbon dioxide, and hormones throughout the body. It plays a crucial role in maintaining homeostasis and overall health. Here is a systematic overview:

1. **Components of the Cardiovascular System**
   - **Heart:** A muscular organ that pumps blood throughout the body.

   - **Blood Vessels:** Network of arteries, veins and capillaries through which blood flows.

   - **Blood:** Fluid that carries oxygen, nutrients, hormones and waste products.

2. **Heart Anatomy**
   - **Chambers:**
     - **Right Atrium:** Receive deoxygenated blood from the body.

- o **Right Ventricle:** Pumps deoxygenated blood to the lungs.

  - o **Left Atrium:** Receives oxygenated blood from the lungs.

  - o **Left Ventricle:** Pumps oxygenated blood to the rest of the body.

- **Valves:**
  - o **Tricuspid Valve:** Between the right atrium and right ventricle.

  - o **Pulmonary Valve:** Between right ventricle and pulmonary artery.

  - o **Mitral Valve:** Between left atrium and left ventricle.

  - o **Aortic Valve:** Between left ventricle and aorta.

3. **Type of Blood Vessels:**
   - **Arteries:** Carry oxygenated blood away from the heart.
     - o **Aorta:** The largest artery, branches out to distribute blood to the body.

     - o **Pulmonary Arteries:** Carry deoxygenated blood to the lungs.

   - **Veins:** Carry deoxygenated blood back to heart.
     - o **Superior and Inferior Vena Cava:** Large veins that brings deoxygenated blood from the body to the right atrium.

- ○ **Pulmonary Veins:** Carry oxygenated blood from lungs to the left atrium.

- • **Capillaries:** Tiny blood vessels where the exchange of gases, nutrients and waste occurs between blood and tissues.

The Heart and Large Blood Vessels

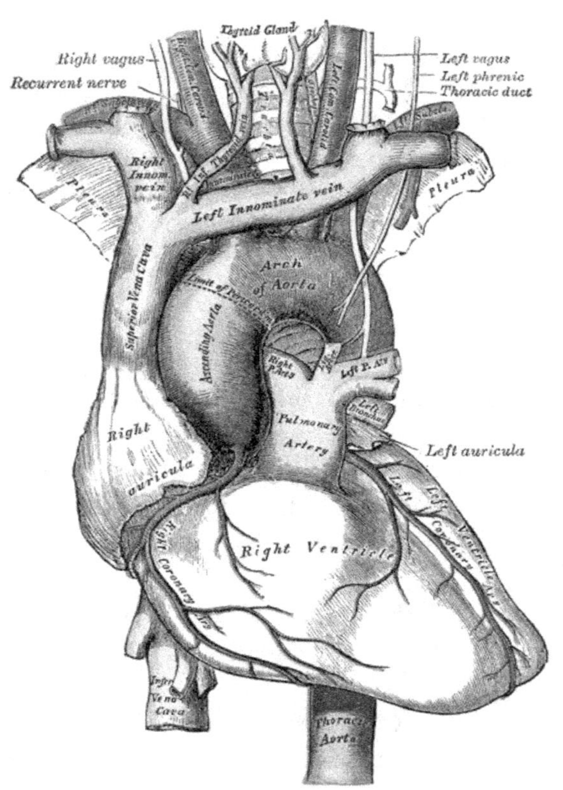

Source: Henry Vandyke Carter / Henry Gray /

Wikimedia Commons

4. **Blood Flow Pathway:**
   - Deoxygenated blood enters the right atrium via the superior and inferior vena cava.

   - Blood flows into right ventricle through the tricuspid valve.

   - The right ventricle pumps blood to the lungs via the pulmonary artery.

   - Oxygenated blood returns to the left atrium through the pulmonary veins.

   - Blood flows into the left ventricle through the mitral valve.

   - The left ventricles pumps blood into the aorta, which distributes it to the rest of the body.

5. **Function of the Cardiovascular System**
   - **Transportation:** Delivers oxygen, nutrients, hormones and removes waste products.

   - **Protection:** The blood contains white blood cells and antibodies that defend against pathogens.

   - **Regulation:** Helps maintain body temperature, Ph balance and fluid balance.

6. **Cardiac Cycle:**
   - **Systole:** Contraction phase where blood is pumped out of the chambers.

   - **Diastole:** Relaxation phase where chambers fill with blood.

Blood Oxygenation in the Pulmonary and Systemic Circulation

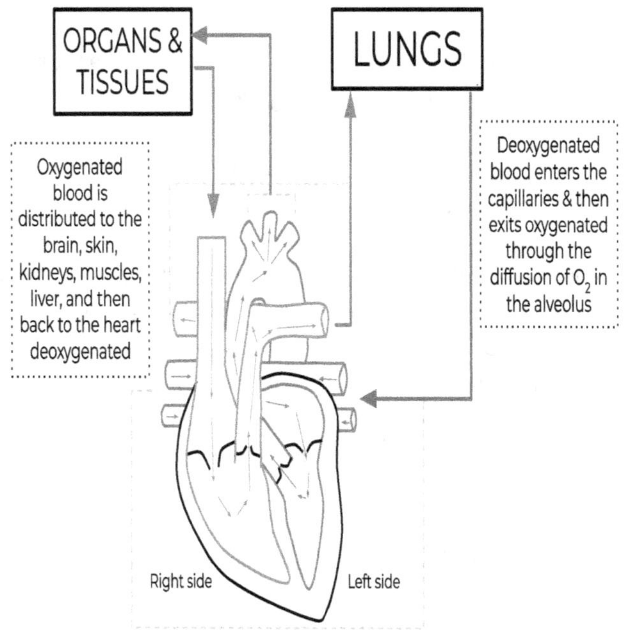

Source: Sasha River Santilla / Wikimedia Commons

7. **Blood Pressure:**
   - **Systolic Blood Pressure:** Pressure during the contraction of the heart.

   - **Diastolic Pressure:** Pressure during relaxation of the heart.

   - Blood pressure is typically measured as systolic/diastolic (e.g. normal B.P. 120/80 mm Hg).

8. Cardiovascular Health
   - Common Conditions: Hypertension, atherosclerosis, coronary artery disease, heart attack and stroke.

   - Preventive Measures: Regular exercise, balanced diet, avoiding smoking and managing stress.

The systemic overview provides a foundational understanding of the cardiovascular system and its essential functions in the body.

(B) What Type of Heart Diseases are Mainly Prevalent in Postmenopausal Women due to Hormonal Changes

Postmenopausal women face increased risk of developing cardiovascular diseases (CVD) due to hormonal changes, especially the decline in estrogen levels. Estrogen is having protective effect on CVS in Pre-menopause. Here is a systematic enumeration of the most common cardiovascular diseases affecting postmenopausal women.

1. **Coronary Artery Disease (CAD)**
   - **Description:** CAD is characterized by the narrowing or the blockage of the coronary arteries due to atherosclerosis, which reduces blood flow to the heart muscle.

   - **Cause:** The drop in estrogen level post-menopause accelerates plaque build-up in the arteries, increasing the risk of heart attacks.

   - **Symptoms:** Chest pain (angina), shortness of breath, fatigue, and heart attack.

   - **Impact:** It is the leading cause of death in postmenopausal women.

2. **Hypertension (High Blood Pressure)**
   - **Description:** Hypertension occurs when the force of blood against the artery wall is consistently too high.

- **Cause:** Postmenopausal hormonal changes lead to increased blood pressure due to stiffening of arteries and weight gain.

- **Symptoms:** Often asymptomatic, but may cause headaches, vision changes and chest pain when severe.

- **Impact:** A major risk factor for other cardiovascular diseases, such as stroke and heart failure.

3. **Heart Failure**
   - **Description:** A condition where the heart is unable to pump blood effectively to meet the body's needs.

   - **Cause:** Coronary artery disease, hypertension and previous heart attacks are common causes of heart failure in postmenopausal women.

   - **Symptoms:** Shortness of breath, swelling in legs, fatigue and fluid buildup in the lungs.

   - **Impact:** It is more common in postmenopausal women due to the cumulative effects of cardiovascular risk factors over time.

4. **Stroke**
   - **Description:** A stroke occurs when blood flow to the brain is interrupted, either by a clot (ischemic stroke).

- **Cause:** Postmenopausal women are at higher risk due to increased blood pressure, diabetes and atrial fibrillation.

- **Symptoms:** Sudden weakness or numbness in the face, arms or legs, difficulty in speaking, vision problems and confusion.

- **Impact:** Stroke is the leading cause of disability and death in postmenopausal women.

5. **Atherosclerosis**
   - **Description:** A condition where fatty deposits (plaque) build up inside the arteries, leading to reduced blood flow and increased risk of heart disease.

   - **Cause:** Decline in estrogen accelerates the process of plaque formation in arteries.

   - **Symptoms:** Often asymptomatic until it causes complications like heart attacks or strokes.

   - **Impact:** Atherosclerosis is a major underlying cause of many cardiovascular diseases in postmenopausal women.

6. **Atrial Fibrillation**
   - **Description:** Atrial fibrillation is an irregular and often rapid heart rate that can lead to poor blood flow and increase the risk of stroke.

   - **Cause:** Aging and hormonal changes contribute to the development of atrial fibrillation in postmenopausal women.

- **Symptoms:** Palpitations, dizziness, shortness of breath and fatigue.

- **Impact:** Atrial fibrillation significantly increases the risk of stroke and heart failure in postmenopausal women.

7. **Peripheral Artery Disease (PAD)**
   - **Description:** PAD occurs when the arteries in the limbs (usually the legs) become narrowed or blocked, reducing blood flow.

   - **Cause:** Atherosclerosis and other cardiovascular risk factors like diabetes and hypertension increase the likelihood of PAD in postmenopausal women.

   - **Symptoms:** Leg pain when walking, cramping and numbness or weakness in the legs.

   - **Impact:** PAD increases the risk of heart attacks and strokes.

8. **Hyperlipidemia (High Cholesterol)**
   - **Description:** Hyperlipidemia refers to abnormally high levels of cholesterol or lipids in the blood, which contribute to plaque buildup in arteries.

   - **Cause:** Menopause is associated with adverse changes in cholesterol levels, particularly an increase in LDL cholesterol (bad cholesterol).

   - **Symptoms:** Often asymptomatic until it leads to conditions like CAD or PAD.

- **Impact:** High cholesterol is a significant risk factor for heart attacks and strokes in postmenopausal women.

9. Venous Thromboembolism (VTE)

- **Description:** VTE is a condition in which blood clots form in the vein, often in legs (deep vein thrombosis), and may travel to the lungs (pulmonary embolism).

- **Causes:** Postmenopausal women, especially those undergoing hormone replacement therapy (HRT), have an increased risk of blood clot formation.

- **Symptoms:** Swelling, pain and redness in the legs (for DVT) or sudden shortness of breath and chest pain (for pulmonary embolism).

- **Impact:** VTE can be life-threatening if not treated promptly.

10. Mitral Valve Prolapse (MVP)

- **Description:** A condition in which the valve between the heart's left atrium and left ventricle does not close promptly.

- **Cause:** While MVP can occur at any age, it becomes more noticeable in postmenopausal women due to aging and changes in the cardiovascular system.

- **Symptoms:** Often asymptomatic but may cause palpitations, shortness of breath and chest pain.

- **Impact:** Though usually benign, MVP can increase the risk of arrhythmias and infective endocarditis.

Conclusion

Postmenopausal women face a heightened risk of various cardiovascular diseases due to hormonal changes and other age-related factors. Early detection, lifestyle modifications and appropriate medical interventions are crucial for managing these conditions and improving cardiovascular health in this population.

CHAPTER III: PATHOLOGY AND SYMPTOMATOLOGY OF MENOPAUSE

"Embrace the change,

it's a beginning of a new, vibrant chapter."

(A) Definition of Menopause:

- Menopause is defined by **Stedman** as permanent cessation of menses. An awareness of menopause can be traced from ancient Greeks. In fact, the word menopause is derived from the Greek word meno meaning month and refers to menstrual cycle, while pause meaning to cease or to stop. In other words, menopause literally means cessation of monthly cycles.

- **The World Health Organization (WHO)** has defined natural menopause as the permanent cessation of menses resulting from loss of ovarian follicular activity. Menopause marks the end of reproductive life and natural menopause is the retrospective clinical diagnosis which occurs after 12 consecutive months of amenorrhoea, for which no other pathological cause can be established.

- The menopausal transition is the time before the final menopausal period **(FMP)** and is associated with irregular cycles, hormonal instability and symptoms.

(B) Pathophysiology of Menopause Transition:

- **Biology of ovarian aging:**

In the human ovary, there is a continuous and progressive decline in the number of follicles from foetal life onwards. From several million follicles present at birth, less than a thousand remain at menopause. The loss cannot be accounted for by ovulation alone. Because the reproductive span of 30-35 years in a woman can only account for a loss of 350-450 ovarian follicles through ovulation. Their disappearance is also related to a loss of oocytes and surrounding granulosa and theca cells of the ovarian follicles that occur continuously through a process of follicular atresia. In every cycle, from a recruited pool of growing follicles, only one dominant follicle is selected, the rest undergoing atresia. It is clear from several studies **(Block 1952, Gougeon 1984, Gosden 1985, Richardson et al 1987)** that serum gonadotropins mainly follicular stimulating hormone (FSH) are responsible for accelerating the pace of follicular atresia leading to the depletion of stock and subsequent menopause.

- **Menopause Markers (Hormonal Changes during menopause transition):**

The transition from the ovulatory cycles to the menopausal state is usually not an instantaneous event. Rather it is a series of hormonal clinical alterations that reflect declining ovarian function. Menopause is diagnosed retrospectively by history. Markers for diagnosis of menopause are preferably restricted for use in special situations and for fertility issues.

- ➢ **FSH** > 10 IU/L is indicative of declining ovarian function.

- ➢ **FSH** > 20 IU/L is diagnostic of ovarian failure in the perimenopausal age group with vasomotor symptoms (VMS) even in the absence of complete cessation of menses.

- ➢ **FSH** > 40 IU/L done 2 months apart is diagnostic of menopause.

- ➢ **FSH** rise precedes the LH rise.

- ➢ **FSH** is a diagnostic marker of ovarian failure while **LH** is not.

- ➢ **LH** measurement is not necessary to make a diagnosis of menopause.

- ➢ 1 - 3 years after menopause, serum **LH** rises by **3 folds** while **FSH** by **10 - 20 folds.** Rise in serum **LH** level is less pronounced than serum **FSH** level because **LH** has a shorter half-life period and has no specific negative peptide. **(FSH has a specific negative feedback peptide called Inhibin.)**

- ➢ **Postmenopausal serum estradiol level falls and it is < 20 pg/ml at menopause.** (Premenopausal level of serum estradiol varies from 40 -400 pg/ml).

- ➢ **AMH** and **Inhibin** levels are low or undetectable at menopause. Inhibin is a polypeptide that is secreted by granulosa cells, it has both paracrine and endocrine functions. At the central level inhibin exerts a negative feedback effect and reduces the pituitary secretion of FSH. At the ovarian level its paracrine function is to prevent folliculogenesis of other follicles. An increasing level of serum FSH during early follicular phase and a decline in circulating levels of inhibin and estradiol are the first indications of age-related acceleration of follicular depletion. Serum inhibin during the early follicular phase showed a significant decline in women of 45-49 years of age as compared to those aged below 45 years **(McLachlan et.al. 1987-88).**

> On transvaginal ultrasound the antral follicular count is low and ovarian volume is also reduced.

- **Estrogen/Testosterone Shift in Menopausal Women and other related factors:**

During menopause, significant hormonal changes occur in women's body, particularly involving estrogen and testosterone. This Estrogen/Testosterone shift has profound effect on both physical and mental health.

o **Estrogen Decline:** Normal serum estradiol level in women in reproductive age group is 40 – 400 pg/ml depending up on the stage of menstrual cycle. Estrogen is a key hormone in female sexual health. It is responsible for maintaining the health of vaginal tissues, promoting lubrication and supporting the overall sexual response cycle. Estradiol level in postmenopausal women is below 20 pg/ml. After menopause, ovaries no longer produce estrogen. Instead, in small amounts it is produced in a number of extra-gonadal sites such as kidney, adipose tissue, skin and brain. Unlike ovarian synthesized estrogen, which is released into the blood stream, estrogen synthesized within these extra-gonadal sites mostly acts locally at the site of synthesis and functions as a paracrine and/or intracrine factor to maintain important tissue specific functions.

- **Impact on Body:**
  - ✓ **Vasomotor Symptoms:** The decline in estrogen is responsible for common menopausal symptoms such as hot flashes and night sweats.

  - ✓ **Bone Health:** Reduced estrogen levels lead to decreased bone density, increasing the risk of osteoporosis.

  - ✓ **Cardiovascular Health:** Estrogen has protective effects on the heart and blood vessels; its decline can lead to an increased risk of cardiovascular diseases.

  - ✓ **Mental Health:** Estrogen influence neurotransmitter systems that regulate mood and cognitive functions. Its decrease can lead to symptoms such as depression, anxiety and cognitive decline.

- **Relative Increase in Testosterone:** While testosterone levels also decline during menopause, the decrease is more gradual compared to estrogen. As a result, there is a relative increase in androgen-to-estrogen ratio. This shift can lead to noticeable changes in a woman's body.

- **Effect of the Estrogen / Testosterone Shift:**
  - ✓ **Androgenic Symptoms:** The relative increase in testosterone can cause symptoms

such as thinning scalp hair, increased facial hairs and a deeper voice.

- ✓ **Libido Changes:** Testosterone plays a role in sexual desire, and the hormonal shift during menopause can lead to changes in libido, with some women experiencing a decrease and others in increase in sexual interest.

- ✓ **Muscle Mass:** Testosterone helps maintain muscle mass, so while overall muscle mass may decline with aging, the relative increase in testosterone can help in preserving it to some extent

- ○ **Overall Impact:**
  The estrogen/testosterone shift during menopause contribute to a range of physical and mental health changes. The decline in estrogen is primarily responsible for the more commonly recognised symptoms of menopause, such as hot flashes, mood swings and increased risk of osteoporosis and cardiovascular issues. Meanwhile the relative increase in sexual function, body function, and the emergence of androgenic symptoms.

- **Changes in cycle length and menstrual bleeding**: Women aged 18-24 years have an average follicular phase length of 15 ± 2 days, but those aged 40 -44 years have an average length of $10 + 2$ days, which tends to shorten the menstrual cycle. Thus, menstrual cycle length may shorten before it lengthens as women progress through the transition. **(Trealar et. al. 1967)**

One hallmark of the menopause transition is a change in bleeding pattern, **Van Voorhis and et. al**. has studied hormonal pattern and menstrual bleeding pattern in a large sub cohort of the **SWAN** participants aged 42-52 years. They found that 20% of all cycles during the time were an ovulatory. They also noted that short cycle lengths (<21 days) were common early in menopause transition whereas long cycle intervals (> 36 days) were associated with late menopause transition.

(C)Age at Menopause:

- The menopause transition most often begins between ages 45 and 55 years. The average age at menopause of an Indian woman is 46.2 years, much less than western woman (51 years).

- From available Indian data it is hypothesized that an early age at menopause in Indian women (46.2 years) predisposes them to chronic health disorders a decade earlier than the Caucasians having late age at menopause (51 years).

- It is reported that osteoporotic fractures occur 10-20 years earlier in Indians as compared to Caucasians.

- The first myocardial infarction (MI) attack occurs in 4.4% of Asian women at a younger age than in European women.

- In India, type II diabetes occurs a decade earlier than the Caucasians.

- Breast cancer is the most common cancer in Indian women and the incidence peaks before the age of 50 years.

As the women approach their mid-forties, many women find themselves looking for signs of menopause and trying to figure out when it will begin for them. Most women reach menopause between the ages of 45 and 55 years. But as every woman is unique, age at menopause may also differ due to underlying conditions.

- **Genetic factors:**
  Research has conclusively shown that there is a strong link between menopause and genetics. There are approximately 50% chances that a woman will become menopausal at the same age as her mother or within a few years of that age. However, this may not always be the case.

- **Ethnicity:**
  Studies have conclusively revealed that the average menopausal age for Caucasian women in the UK and USA is around 51 years, while in Indians it is 46.2 yrs. The reason for these variations is that women of different ethnicities often have different levels of estrogenic activity.

- **Smoking:**
  Smoking has been found to be the number one modifiable lifestyle factor relating to early menopause. Polycyclic aromatic hydrocarbons found in cigarette smoke are toxic to ovarian follicles. These chemicals can cause premature loss of follicles leading to early onset of menopause.
  Smoking can lead to faster breakdown of oestrogen in the liver which in turn results in an earlier decline in oestrogen level.

- **Body Mass Index (BMI):**
  A study conducted by Australian University has shown that women who are underweight or have a low BMI are more likely to enter menopause early,

while women who are overweight or have high BMI are more likely to experience a late menopause. This is due to the fact that oestrogen is stored in fat cells.

- **Parity**:
  Nulliparous women may experience an earlier menopause while multiparty or a late first pregnancy may result in a later onset.

- **Other factors include:**
  Women with bilateral oophorectomy, exposure to radiotherapy or chemotherapy in premenopausal age experience early induced menopause.

- Use of oral contraceptives may delay the onset.

Is there a menopause age calculator?

All factors discussed above could help women to determine the appropriate age at menopause but there is no definite test to predict it. In a nutshell AMH levels indicate the number of follicles present in the ovaries and unlike FSH levels, AMH levels do not fluctuate with phases in menstrual cycles, which means that they can be used to determine the extent of ovarian reserve and thereby the approximate age at which menopause will occur.

(D)Terminologies in Relation to Menopause:

- **Natural Menopause:**
  It is recognised to have occurred after 12 months of amenorrhoea for which there are no obvious pathological causes.

- **Premenopause:**
  It is often used to refer to the entire reproductive period up to the final menstrual period (FMP).

- **Perimenopause:**
  It is the period immediately before 2 - 3 years and 1 year after FMP. It may last up to 3 - 5 yrs. The characteristics are:
  - Increasing serum FSH levels
  - Significantly reduced fertility
  - Erratic menstrual periods
  - Onset of menstrual symptoms

  (The term is used interchangeably with menopause transition.)

- **Climacteric:**
  It is interchangeably used with perimenopause and menopause transition. When associated with symptoms, it is called climacteric syndrome.

- **Postmenopause:**
  It is the span of life dating from the final menstrual period onwards regardless of whether the menopause was spontaneous or iatrogenic.

- **Premature Ovarian Insufficiency (POI):**
  Premature ovarian Insufficiency has replaced the term premature menopause. POI is described as amenorrhoea due to loss of ovarian function before the

age of 40 years. It is a state of female hypergonadotrophic hypogonadism. Its incidence is 1%. It can manifest as primary amenorrhoea with onset before menarche or secondary amenorrhoea with onset after the establishment of natural menses. Criteria for diagnosis of POI as per ***European Society of Human Reproduction and Embryology (ESHRE 2015) is 'Elevated FSH levels > 25 IU/L on two occasions > 4 weeks apart'.***

- **Early Menopause**:
  It is the time span between the spontaneous or iatrogenic menopause occurring between 40 years of age and the accepted typical age of menopause for a given population (between 40 and 46.2 years in Indian population). Incidence is 5%.

- **Delayed Menopause:**
  It is not well defined but may be important in terms of increased problems associated with hyperestrogenism. It is two SDs above from the natural average age of menopause in a given population. In India, we may consider it to be 54 years or more.

- **Postmenopausal Bleeding (PMB):**
  It is the bleeding which occurs 12 months after the last menstrual period. However, it is recommended that any vaginal bleeding that occurs 6 months after the last menstrual period should be investigated.

- **Induced Menopause/Surgical Menopause**:
  It is the cessation of menses due to bilateral oophorectomy or iatrogenic ablation of ovarian function or hysterectomy.

(C)Symptoms of Menopause:

- About 20% of women have no symptoms at all, while 60% have mild to moderate symptoms. The remaining 20% have severe symptoms that interfere with their daily life.

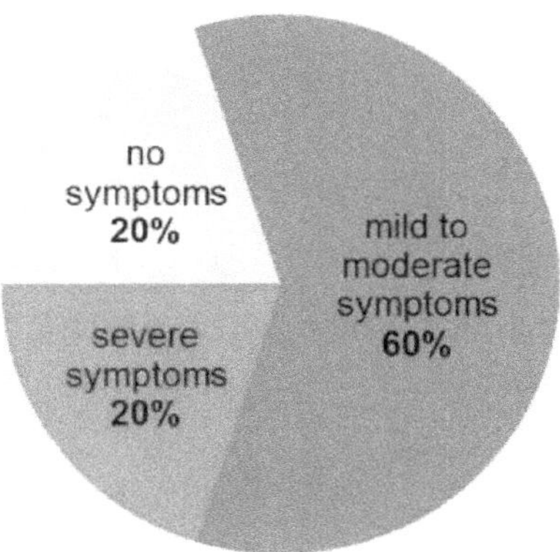

- Menopausal symptoms can be influenced by different factors, for example, your stage of life and general health and wellbeing.

- The biology and symptomatology of menopause is blurred due to its relationship to the underlying aging process.

- Vasomotor, urogenital symptoms and irregular menstrual periods are typically linked with serum oestrogen levels.

- Long term effects on bone and heart have been related to oestrogen deficiency.

- Many other symptoms like muscle and joint pain, vertigo, mood changes, depression, insomnia, nervousness have been associated with menopause but are not necessarily due to decrease in oestrogen levels.

- Many symptoms start during perimenopause and can continue into postmenopause. Australian studies show that some women experience symptoms like hot flashes and night sweats well into their 60s.

Physical Symptoms:

Physical symptoms may include:

- Irregular periods
- Hot flashes
- Night sweats
- Sleep problems
- Sore breasts
- Itchy, crawly or dry skin
- Exhaustion and fatigue
- Dry vagina
- Loss of sex drive (libido)
- Headaches or migraine
- Aches and pains
- Bloating
- Urinary problems
- Weight gains due to androgen-oestrogen ratio shift and low BMR.

Emotional symptoms may include:

- Feeling irritable or frustrated
- Feeling anxious
- Difficulty in concentrating
- Forgetfulness
- Mood swings

Symptoms and Disorders in Relation to Age and Menopause:

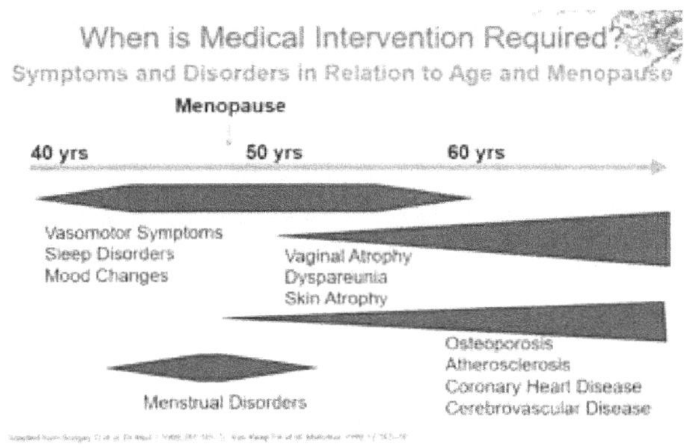

Source: Bungay G, et al. Br Med J 1980; 281: 181 - 3;

Van Keep PA, et al. Maturities 1990; 12:163-70.

> *The immediate symptoms of menopause transition are irregular periods, hot flashes, night sweats, sleep and mood disturbances, joint and muscle pain, vaginal dryness and low sexual desire which generally resolve over a while in mild cases.*

> *Genitourinary symptoms appear in the early postmenopausal period and may worsen over some time if not treated.*

> *The long-term consequences of menopause affect bone and cardiovascular health which worsen with aging.*

Overview of Cardiovascular Risk in Postmenopausal Women

Postmenopausal women have an increased risk of cardiovascular disease (CVD) due to hormonal changes, especially **due to the decline in estrogen levels**, which plays a protective role in maintaining vascular health in premenopausal years.

Estrogen deficiency is associated with:

- Adverse changes in lipid profiles

- Endothelial dysfunction and

- An increased risk of atherosclerosis

- Weight Gain: Many women experience weight gain during menopause due to redistribution of fat around abdomen. This can increase the risk of metabolic syndrome.

- Insulin Resistance: Menopause may contribute to insulin resistance, increasing the risk of diabetes.

- Mental Health: Hormonal changes during menopause can lead to mood swing, irritability and depression. Night sweats and hot flashes can disturb sleep.

leading to a **higher incidence of heart attacks and strokes.**

Details we will be discussing in the next chapters.

Recent data from longitudinal studies have shown that menopause related factors, such as earlier age at menopause (< 45 years), surgical menopause, and POI (Premature Ovarian Insufficiency < 40 years of age) are associated with higher CVD risk. Type 2 Diabetes may further augment the risk, particularly in black women.

CHAPTER IV: RISK FACTORS FOR CARDIOVASCULAR HEALTH

"Menopause isn't just a life change, it's reminder for women to take charge of their heart health and embrace new chapter of wellness."

(A)Key Points:

- Cardiovascular disease (CVD) is the leading cause of death in United States and worldwide.

- Cardiovascular disease is number one killer in postmenopausal women, cancer being second.

- Women can develop heart disease at any age, but the risk increases after menopause, usually after the age of 55 years.

- It is assumed that estrogen is cardio protective in premenopausal women.

- Epidemiological evidence has shown that menopausal transition is associated with a higher prevalence of CVD risk factors such as central obesity, atherogenic dyslipidemia, insulin resistance and arterial hypertension.

- Menopause is often a turning point for women's health worldwide. Cardio metabolic changes can manifest at the menopause transition, superimposing the effect of ageing onto the risk of cardiovascular disease.

- **Menopause can be considered as a "Biological Marker of cardiovascular disease".**

- While average age for heart attack is 64.5 years for men and 70.3 years for women, nearly 20% of those who die of heart disease are under the age of 65 years.

- Cardiovascular diseases which are the leading cause of death in postmenopausal women include:

  o Coronary heart disease or
    Ischemic heart disease or
    Atherosclerotic heart disease or
    Atherosclerotic cardiovascular disease

  o Stroke and

  o Venous thromboembolism

- Coronary artery disease is the most common type of heart disease and the cause of heart attacks in women.

- Studies strongly suggest that there is association of increase in cardiovascular events after menopause, distinct from other risk factors common to both genders.

- Additionally, there are some nontraditional women-specific risk factors such as pregnancy complications, PCOD, autoimmune diseases and age at menarche.

(B) Traditional Risk Factors for Cardiovascular Disease Common to Both Genders:

The genesis of cardiovascular disease is multifactorial. The factors contributing to the development of CVD starts at the intrauterine stage, which is called the '**Barkers Hypothesis.**' The other factors are:

1. **Biological Factors:**
   - **Age:**
   Increased risk as age advances in both genders.

   - **Gender:**
   Postmenopausal women have a higher risk than premenopausal women due to the drop in estrogen level.

   - **Family History:**
   A family history of cardiovascular diseases increases the risk.

   - **Menopause:**
   Natural or surgical menopause is linked to an increased risk of CVD due to hormonal changes.

2. **Lifestyle Factors:**
   - **Smoking:**
   Active smoking or exposure to secondhand smoke significantly increase cardiovascular risk.

   - **Physical Inactivity:**
   Sedentary Lifestyles contributes to obesity, high blood pressure, and cholesterol issues.

- **Unhealthy Diet:**
  Diets high in saturated fats, cholesterol and sodium increases the risk of heart disease.

- **Excessive Alcohol Consumption:**
  Heavy drinking can lead to high blood pressure, heart failure and stroke.

- **Obesity:**
  Excess body weight, especially abdominal obesity, is a major risk factor for heart disease.

3. **Medical Conditions:**

- High Blood Pressure (Hypertension):
  One of the leading causes of cardiovascular disease.

- High Cholesterol Level:
  Elevated levels of LDL (bad cholesterol) and low levels of HDL (good) cholesterol.

- **Diabetes:**
  Increased blood sugar levels can damage blood vessels and nerves that control the heart.

- **Metabolic Syndrome:**
  A cluster of conditions including high blood pressure, high blood sugar, excess body fat, and abnormal cholesterol levels.

- **Chronic Kidney Disease:**
  Linked with higher cardiovascular risks due to its impact and blood pressure and fluid balance.

4. **Hormonal Factors:**
   - **Low Estrogen Levels:**
     After menopause, the reduction in estrogen can lead to adverse changes in blood vessel walls and cholesterol levels.

   - **Hormonal Replacement Therapy:**
     Depending on timings, type, and duration; HRT can influence cardiovascular risk in various ways.

5. **Psychological Factors:**
   - **Stress:**
     Chronic stress contributes to high blood pressure and other cardiovascular risks.

   - **Depression and Anxiety:**
     Mental health conditions can negatively impact heart health through lifestyle changes and physiological responses.

6. **Sleep-Related Factors:**
   - **Sleep Apnea:**
     Obstructive sleep apnea increases blood pressure and put strain on cardiovascular system.

   - **Poor Sleep Quality:**
     Inadequate or disturbed sleep is linked to an increased risk of hypertension, obesity, and diabetes.

It is important to note that these factors can interact with each other and with an individual's genetic predisposition, making it crucial to address and manage them to reduce the risk of cardiovascular disease. Regular check-ups with healthcare professionals can help identify and manage these risk factors effectively.

In this book we are not going to discuss the traditional risk factors in detail common to both genders as mentioned above. **But here, we are interested more in women- specific risk factors which are contributing to CVD risk in women in addition to traditional risk factors common to both genders.**

(C) Gender Differences in Cardiovascular Disease: (Why women are at greater risk for CVD?)

- **Prevalence of Cardiovascular Disease:**
Prevalence of CVD can vary between males and females and may be influenced by age. Generally, men have a higher incidence of CVD in younger ages compared with women. This is partly attributed to the cardioprotective effects of estrogen in premenopausal women. However, after menopause, the risk of CVD in women increases and eventually catches up to that of men.

- **CVD Research Predominantly Focused on Women:**
It is important to acknowledge that historically, CVD research has predominantly focused on men. This has led to a knowledge gap in understanding the unique aspects of CVD in women. As a result, symptoms and risk factors specific to women may be underdiagnosed and undertreated. It's taken more than a decade for doctors to realize that more women are affected due to CVD events in postmenopausal women.

  - **Initial Perception of CVD as a Male Disease:**
  For decades, heart disease was widely considered a condition that primarily affected men. This perception likely stemmed from the fact that men often develop CVD at a younger age than women. As a result, researchers and clinicians concentrated their efforts on understanding and treating CVD in men, overlooking

its impact on women, particularly postmenopausal women.

- o **Gender Bias in Medical Research:**
  Historically medical research, including clinical trials, often excluded women or included them in significantly smaller numbers. Women are frequently left out of studies due to concerns about hormonal fluctuations affecting study outcomes, the potential effects on pregnancy, and perceived differences in drug metabolism. This male- centric research design resulted in a lack of data on how CVD manifests differently in women.

- o **Difference in Symptoms and Presentation:**
  With men, heart disease typically manifests itself through the classic symptoms such as crushing or squeezing chest pain or tightness in the chest. Women on the other hand may occasionally present as chest pain but most often present with shortness of breath, pain in neck, jaw, throat, and upper abdomen or back. Women tends to have a lot of vague symptoms such as just being tired, not being able to say what's wrong with them. On the top of that 64% of women who die suddenly of coronary heart disease have no previous symptoms. And that's why succumb to death due to CVD without being treated in time. These differences in symptom presentation led to underdiagnosis and misinterpretation of women's symptoms, further reinforcing the notion that heart disease was a male dominated issue.

- o **Focus on Reproductive in Women Health Research:**
  Much of the historical research on women's health concentrated on reproductive health, including pregnancy, contraception and menopause. This narrow

focus meant that conditions like CVD, which affect both men and women, were not prioritized within women-specific health research.

- o **Delayed Recognition of CVD risk in Women:**
  It was only relatively recently recognized that CVD is the leading cause of death in women, particularly postmenopausal women. This delayed recognition contributed to a lack of dedicated research efforts to explore CVD's unique risk factors, presentation, and outcomes in women.

  This historical male focus in CVD research has resulted in gap in understanding how cardiovascular diseases affect women differently, leading to calls for more gender-specific research and tailored healthcare practices in recent years.

- **Smaller Arteries in Women Than Men:**
  Anatomical and physiological differences between men and women, which significantly impact the development, diagnosis and treatment of coronary artery disease (CAD) in women. Here is a more detailed breakdown of these points.

- o **Smaller Arteries in Women:**
  Women generally have smaller coronary arteries than men. This difference can influence the progression and presentation of coronary artery disease. In women coronary artery disease often develops more diffusely rather than as large localized blockages. As a result, traditional diagnostic methods like angiograms, which are designed to detect larger, more obvious blockages in the main coronary arteries, might miss the subtler, diffuse narrowing often seen in women.

- o **Microvascular Dysfunction:**
  Women are more prone to microvascular dysfunction, a condition that affects the tiny blood vessels in the heart. In microvascular disease, the smaller branches of the coronary arteries can become dysfunctional, reducing blood flow and causing symptoms similar to those of CVD. This issue is complex because it doesn't present as clear blockages, which make it harder to diagnose using conventional methods like coronary angiography.

- o **Challenges in Diagnosis:**
  Since angiograms primarily identify blockages in large coronary arteries, they may not always detect the diffuse or microvascular disease more commonly found in women. This diagnostic limitation can lead to women experiencing chest pain or other cardiovascular symptoms despite "normal" angiogram results. As a result, their conditions may go undiagnosed or be misinterpreted as non-cardiac issue, contributing to proper treatment.

- o **Treatment Challenges:**
  Because of diffuse nature of coronary disease in women and the involvement of microvascular dysfunction, standard treatments of CAD, such as stent placement or bypass surgery, are often less effective. Women with microvascular disease may require alternative treatment approaches, such as medications to improve microvascular function or therapies tailored to their unique disease patterns.

These anatomical and physiological differences underscore the need for a gender-specific approach to cardiovascular disease. A greater emphasis on understanding microvascular disease, combined with adjustments in diagnostic techniques, is crucial to better manage and treat heart disease in women. Additionally increased awareness among healthcare professionals about these gender differences can lead to more accurate diagnosis and personalized treatments, ultimately improving outcomes for women with cardiovascular disease.

- Studies have shown that endogenous estrogen during reproductive period delays manifestation of atherosclerotic disease in women. And that may be the reason that CVD develops 7 – 10 years later in women than men and still the number one cause of death in women after the age of 65 years.

- **WISE Study (Women's Ischemic Syndrome Evaluation Study),** shows that young women with premature ovarian insufficiency (POI) have 7-fold increase in coronary artery disease risk. Again, they have approximately 2 years lower life expectancy compared with women with a normal menopause.

- **Obesity, another traditional risk factor is more prevalent in women than in men. Obesity has independently shown to be associated with increased risk of CVD.**
  - According to the **National Health and Nursing Examination Survey (NHNES) in 2013**, among 37.7% of adults aged 20 years or older who are classified as obese, 40.4% were women as against 35% men.

  - **Framingham Heart Study** found obesity to increase relative risk of CVD by 64% in women compared with 46% in men.

  - Central obesity with an increase in visceral fat occurs more frequently after menopause in women, with a higher risk of comorbid risk factors and components of metabolic syndrome in women compared with ageing men.

- **The risk of diabetes on CVD is different in women than in men. Diabetic women are disproportionately affected.**

  o Mortality for diabetic women is an estimated 2.1 million versus 1.8 million in diabetic men, and majority of these deaths are cardiovascular in nature.

  o In women with DM, there is a 1.81-fold increased risk of death from ischemic heart disease compared with women without DM, while diabetic men have 1.48-fold increased risk when compared with nondiabetic men.

  o Risk of heart failure is 5-fold higher in diabetic women as compared with nondiabetic, while in diabetic men the risk is 2-fold as against nondiabetic men.

- **Hypertension** is another well-established risk factor for CVD and the leading cause of cardiovascular mortality worldwide. Women with hypertension have a higher population-adjusted cardiovascular mortality when compared with men and are less likely to be treated by guideline-directed blood pressure goals.

- **At younger ages (< 50 years) smoking is more deleterious in women than in men, resulting in increased risk of a first acute myocardial infarction relatively more in women than in men.**
Gender-specific impact of smoking on cardiovascular health, particularly in younger women (< 50 years of age)

Research indicates that smoking is indeed more deleterious in women under the age of 50 compared to their male counterparts, especially in terms of increasing a risk of a first myocardial infarction (heart attack). Here is a deeper look at why smoking may pose a greater risk for younger women:

o **Heightened Biological Sensitivity:**
Women, particularly those under 50, seem to have a heightened biological sensitivity to the harmful effects of smoking. This increased sensitivity may be due to in part to how smoking interacts with estrogen, a hormone that typically offers some degree of cardiovascular protection. Smoking accelerates the decline in estrogen levels, reducing this protective effect and leading to an increased risk of cardiovascular events such as heart attack.

o **Greater Relative Risk:**
Studies have shown that women who smoke have a proportionately higher relative risk of developing coronary artery disease and suffering a first myocardial infarction compared to male smokers. While smoking significantly increases heart disease risk for both sexes, the relative risk is amplified in women. For example, while male smokers might have a 2-fold increased risk of heart attack, female smokers can have a 3-fold or even higher risk.

o **Impact on Vascular Health:**
Smoking contributes to endothelial dysfunction, the narrowing of blood vessels, and increased atherosclerosis (plaques buildup in arteries). Women's arteries, being generally smaller, are more vulnerable to these effects. Thus, the vascular changes induced by smoking can have a more pronounced impact on blood flow in women, increasing their likelihood of

developing acute cardiovascular events at a younger age.

o **Interaction With Other Risk Factors:**
Younger women who smoke are often affected by other compounding risk factors, such as oral contraceptive use. The combination of oral contraceptives significantly increases the risk of thrombotic events, including heart attacks and strokes, in women. The interaction creates a dangerous synergy that heightens the cardiovascular risks associated with smoking more dramatically in women than in men.

o **Increased Clotting Tendency:**
Smoking has been shown to increase the tendency for blood clotting (thrombogenesis). Women, due to hormonal factors and the influence of estrogen, might have a naturally higher baseline risk of clotting. When combined with pro-thrombotic effects of smoking, this can lead to an increased likelihood of acute myocardial infarction, particularly in younger age group.

The heightened risk of acute myocardial infarction in younger women smokers underscores the importance of targeted smoking cessation efforts. For women under 50, quitting smoking can significantly reduce their elevated cardiovascular risk, potentially bringing it closer to that of non-smokers. This gender-specific difference in smoking-related risk also calls for greater awareness among healthcare providers, who should be proactive in assessing and addressing cardiovascular risk factors in younger female patients who smoke.

- Pregnancy complications such as pre-eclampsia, gestational diabetes and preterm births, autoimmune diseases, PCOD and age at menarche contribute additional risk factors in some women.

(D) Women-Specific Risk Factors for CVD

Gender differences in pathophysiology, prevalence and impact of cardiovascular disease risk factors may explain the high cardiovascular mortality rates in women. **For better understanding women-specific risk factors can be described under 3 headings:**

1. **Estrogen as cardioprotective in premenopausal women.**
2. **Menopause as a risk factor of CVD due to estrogen deficiency.**
3. **Non-traditional risk factors in some women.**

Estrogen as cardioprotective in premenopausal women:

Estrogen has regulatory effect on several metabolic factors such as inflammatory markers, lipids and coagulatory system.

Cardioprotective effect of estrogen through its anti-inflammatory action:

- Estrogen has been found to exhibit anti-inflammatory properties, which can contribute to its cardioprotective effects in the prevention of CVD. Inflammation plays a significant role in the development and progression of cardiovascular disease including atherosclerosis.

- Estrogen has been shown to modulate the immune response and reduce the production of pro-inflammatory molecules in the body. It can inhibit the expression of certain inflammatory markers such as cytokines and adhesion molecules, which are involved in the initiation and progression of inflammation.

- By reducing inflammation, estrogen helps to maintain the integrity of blood vessels and prevent the formation of atherosclerotic plaques. Atherosclerosis is a condition characterized by the accumulation of cholesterol and immune cells in the arterial walls, leading to the narrowing and hardening of blood vessels. Estrogen's anti-inflammatory action can help inhibit the inflammatory process that contribute to the development of atherosclerosis.

- Additionally, estrogen has been shown to promote the production of anti-inflammatory molecules such as interleukin-10 (IL-10), which further helps to counteract inflammation and protect against CVD.

Cardioprotective effect of estrogen through its regulation on lipid profile:

- Estrogen plays a role in regulating lipid profile, specifically by influencing the role of different lipids in the blood stream. It has both direct and indirect effects on lipid metabolism.

- One way estrogen affects lipid profile is by increasing the levels of high-density lipoprotein (HDL-C), often referred to as good cholesterol. HDL-C helps remove LDL-C, often referred as bad cholesterol from blood stream, reducing the risk of plaque buildup in the arteries.

- Estrogen also has indirect effects on lipid metabolism by influencing the activity of enzymes involved in lipid synthesis and breakdown. It can decrease the production of triglycerides, a type of fat found in blood, by inhibiting the enzyme lipoprotein lipase.

- Estrogen promotes and maintains gynecoid body fat distribution.

- Additionally, estrogen can increase the breakdown of LDL-C receptors, which help remove LDL-C from blood stream.

Cardioprotective effect of estrogen through its role in regulating the coagulatory system:

- Estrogen plays a role in regulating the coagulatory system, which is responsible for maintaining the balance between blood clotting and preventing the coagulatory system through various mechanisms.

- One way, estrogen influences the coagulatory system, is by increasing the production of certain clotting factors, such as fibrinogen and Van Willebrand factor. These clotting factors are essential for the formation of clots. Estrogen can also enhance the activity of other clotting factors such as factor VII, VIII and X.

- Additionally, estrogen has been found to decrease the production of certain anticoagulant proteins such as protein S and antithrombin III.

Cardioprotective effect of estrogen through Nitric Oxide (NO):

- Estrogen has been found to have a cardioprotective effect through its interaction with nitric oxide. Nitric Oxide plays crucial role in maintaining cardioprotective health. It helps to relax and dilate blood vessels, improving blood flow and reducing the risk of high blood pressure and subsequent CVD.

- Estrogen enhances the production and availability of nitric oxide by stimulating the production of endothelial nitric oxide synthase (eNOS), an enzyme responsible for synthesizing NO in endothelial cells lining the blood vessels. This increased production of nitric oxide helps to maintain the flexibility and health of blood vessels, preventing the development of atherosclerosis and reducing the risk of CVD.

Cardioprotective action of estrogen through its antioxidant effect:

- Antioxidants are substances that help neutralize harmful free radicals in the body, which can cause oxidative stress and damage cells, including those of cardiovascular system.

- Estrogen acts as an antioxidant by directly scavenging free radicals and inhibiting their harmful effects. It can donate an electron to stabilize the free radicals and prevent them in causing damage to cells and tissues. This antioxidant activity helps to reduce oxidative stress and protect CVS from damage.

- Estrogen also stimulates the production of endogenous antioxidants, such as **superoxide dismutase (SOD) and glutathione,** which further enhances its cardioprotective effect. These antioxidants help to neutralize free radicals and maintain the balance between oxidative stress and antioxidant defence in the body.

It is important to note that the mechanisms by which endogenous estrogen is cardioprotective in premenopausal women are complex and not fully understood. Researchers continue to study and explore the various ways in which estrogen protects blood vessels and cardiovascular system as a whole in premenopausal women.

Pathophysiology of CVD in Postmenopausal Women due to Estrogen Deficiency.

Estrogen deficiency in postmenopausal women can increase CVD risk through various mechanisms.

Endothelial Dysfunction:

- Estrogen deficiency can lead to impaired endothelial function, promoting the development of arterial stiffness and hypertension.

- Menopause has shown to be associated with more atherogenic shift in the lipid profile. Estrogen deficiency may result in unfavorable lipid changes disturbing the normal lipid profile, thus increasing the risk of atherosclerosis.

  Menopause related lipid changes are:
  - Increased total cholesterol (> 200 mg/dl)
  - Increased triglycerides (> 150 mg/dl)
  - Increased LDL-C (Bad cholesterol > 100 mg/dl)
  - Increased lipoprotein (a)
  - Decreased HDL-C (Good Cholesterol < 40 mg/dl)

Vasoconstriction:

- Estrogen deficiency can lead to reduced Nitric Oxide (NO) formation resulting in narrowing of blood vessels which promotes further elevating blood pressure.

Abdominal or Visceral Obesity:

- After menopause, there is decrease in estrogen levels, which can lead to a shift in fat distribution. Fat tends to be redistributed from peripheral areas (such as hip and thigh) to the abdominal region. This central or visceral fat is more metabolically active and is associated with a higher risk of various health issues, including cardiovascular disease, type 2 diabetes and metabolic syndrome.

- Visceral fat is different from subcutaneous fat because it surrounds internal organs like liver, pancreas and intestines. It can release inflammatory substances and hormones that affect insulin resistance and overall metabolic health.

Main factors contributing to menopausal changes in body composition

Genetic factors	Hormonal factors	Exogenous factors
		Unhealthy nutrition
Genetic predisposition	Rapid hypoestrogenemia	Low physical activity
Ethnicity	Relative	activity
Epigenetic changes	hyperandrogenemia	Drugs (e.g. steroids,
	Low SHBG levels	insulin)
		Diseases

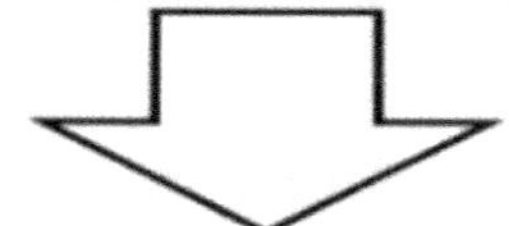

Increase in body weight
Increase and redistribution of fat mass (from gynoid to abdominal obesity)
Decrease in fat-free mass

Metabolic Syndrome:

- Metabolic syndrome is a cluster of conditions that occurs together, increasing the risk of CVD and type 2 diabetes. To diagnose metabolic syndrome, a woman must have at least 3 of the following risk factors.

  - **Central Obesity**
    As per **WHO** criteria waist circumference >80 cm and waist-to-hip ratio > 0.85

  - **High Blood Pressure**
    Elevated blood pressure typically defined as 130/85 mm of Hg and more.

  - **Insulin Resistance**
    Elevated fasting blood sugar levels > 100 mg/dl or more, indicating insulin resistance or prediabetes or frank type 2 diabetes.

  - **High triglycerides**
    >150 mg /dl

  - **Low HDL-C**
    <40 mg /dl

- Each component of metabolic syndrome such as hypertension, dyslipidemia and insulin resistance can independently contribute to the development of CVD.

- The risk factors of metabolic syndrome can interact with each other, further increasing the risk of CVD. For example, insulin resistance can contribute to type 2 DM, hypertension and dyslipidemia, accelerating the development of atherosclerosis and ultimately CVD.

- Metabolic syndrome is associated with chronic low-grade inflammation and increased oxidative stress, which can damage blood vessels and promote atherosclerosis.

Illustration of Atherosclerotic Stages

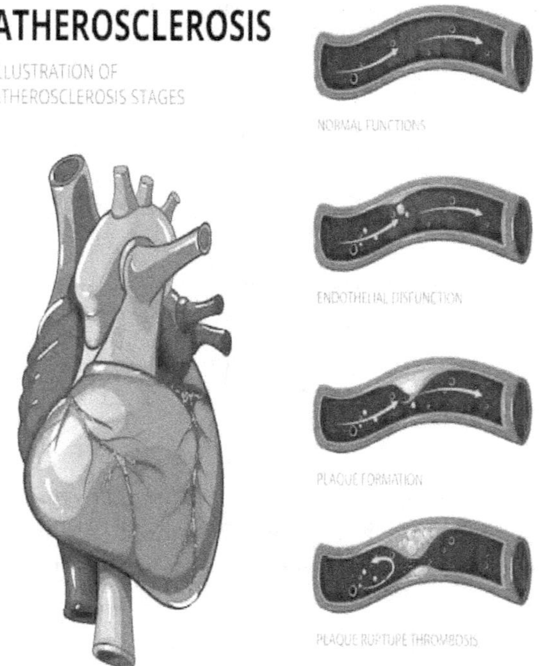

Source: Freepik.com

Fat That Surrounds the Heart is Associated with Increased Risk of CVD.

- Postmenopausal women are at greater risk for heart disease due to a greater volume of a type of fat that surround the heart. Two types of fat that surrounds the heart are epicardial fat and pericardial fat. Epicardial fat covers the heart tissue and is located between the visceral pericardium and the myocardium and covers about 80% of heart surface. Epicardial fat is the energy source for the heart. While pericardial fat, is located between the visceral and parietal pericardial planes, and attached to the external side of the parietal pericardium. There is no protective function of this fat. In fact, the literature review showed that:

    o The greater pericardial fat volume in postmenopausal women was not only linked to lower levels of estradiol, but it is also associated with a greater risk of coronary artery calcification, which is an early sign of heart disease.

    o Among the study participants, 60% increase in pericardial fat was associated with a 45% increase in risk of coronary artery calcification in postmenopausal women compared with premenopausal women.

Prothrombotic State:

- Metabolic syndrome is linked to prothrombotic state, meaning higher tendency for blood clot formation which can lead to heart attacks and strokes.

Non-traditional Risk Factors Contributing to CVD in Some Women:

Apart from the traditional risk factors common to both genders and the menopause related risk factors due to estrogen deficiency, there are some additional nontraditional risk factors in some women, thereby increasing the risk of CVD.

Following are some of the Non-traditional Risk Factors. We will navigate them one by one.

1. **Pregnancy complications such as:**
   o Pre-eclampsia/Gestational Hypertension
   o Gestational Diabetes
   o Preterm Pregnancy
   o Multiple Pregnancy Losses

2. **Age at Menarche**

3. **PCOD (Polycystic Ovarian Disease)**

4. **Autoimmune Diseases**

Pregnancy Complications:

- Researchers have shown that women with history of adverse pregnancy outcomes are at increased risk of cardiovascular disease later in life.

- Pregnancy itself is considered to be the challenge to the maternal cardiovascular system. The maternal cardiovascular system goes through several important adaptations during pregnancy. The cardiac output, heart rate and stroke volume increases during pregnancy due to plasma volume expansion and systemic vascular dilatation. These changes may be attributed to the normal pregnancy outcomes in relation to growing fetus and the mother. Majority of the women withstand this **"Physiological Stress"** without any complications.

- In some women, who experience complications, either there is lack of development of above-mentioned physiological changes in relation to cardiovascular disease or they cannot withstand this physiological stress resulting in pregnancy complications. Exact reason is not known as pregnancy complications are again multifactorial. Further research will clarify the things.

- Therefore, it may be assumed that pregnancy may be considered as a **"Physiological Stress Test",** as the stress it places on woman's body may reveal underlying predisposition to CVD later in life that would otherwise remain hidden for many years as per some of the studies.

- ***Care guidelines from the American Heart Association and American College of Obstetrician & Gynecologist** encourage healthcare providers to ask about a women's pregnancy history and to consider above mentioned pregnancy complications for future heart disease. **American College of Obstetricians and gynecologist's guidelines recommend a yearly assessment to check blood pressure, cholesterol, weight and blood sugar levels for women with a history of early onset or recurrent pre-eclampsia.***

Link Between Pre-Eclampsia and the Risk of CVD Later in Life.

Pre-eclampsia is a relatively common complication of pregnancy with prevalence of 3 – 7%. It is the leading cause of morbidity and mortality for a pregnant woman and also has a significant burden on the healthcare system worldwide.

A 2017 systemic review and meta-analysis of 22 studies found that pre-eclampsia is associated with 4-fold increase in future heart failure risk and 2-fold increase in coronary heart disease, stroke and cardiovascular death.

Research studies have found that women who experience gestational hypertension/pre-eclampsia during pregnancy may be at higher risk of developing CVD later in life. The exact reasons for this association are not fully understood, but several factors are believed to play a role. Here are some of the risk factors.

- **Endothelial Dysfunction:**
  Gestational hypertension and pre-eclampsia can cause damage to the lining of blood vessels (endothelium), leading to the impaired vascular function and increasing the risk of atherosclerosis.

- **Chronic Inflammation:**
  Both conditions involve inflammation and oxidative stress, which can contribute to the development of CVD events over time.

- **Insulin Resistance:**
  Gestational hypertension/pre-eclampsia have been linked to insulin resistance, which is a risk factor for type 2 DM and metabolic syndrome further increasing the risk of CVD.

- o **Persistent hypertension (Chronic hypertension):**
  Women who experience gestational hypertension may have a higher likelihood of developing chronic hypertension after giving birth, which is significant risk factor for heart disease.

Link Between Gestational Diabetes and the Risk of CVD Later in Life

Here are some of the risk factors which contribute to increased CVD risk.

GDM affects 4 -7 % of pregnancies.

20-60 % of women will develop type 2 DM later in life within 5-10 years of index pregnancy.

GDM is associated with 2-fold risk of future cardiovascular events, with the risk being apparent within 10 years after pregnancy.

Here are some of the key factors:

- o **Insulin Resistance:**
  Gestational diabetes is characterized by insulin resistance, where the body cells do not respond effectively to insulin. The condition may persist after pregnancy and can lead to the development of type 2 DM, which is a significant risk factor for CVD.

- o **Atherosclerosis:**
  Insulin resistance and chronically high blood sugar levels can promote the development of atherosclerosis.

Link Between Preterm Delivery and Risk of CVD Later in Life

Preterm delivery refers to giving birth before 37 weeks of gestation and is associated with certain maternal health implications including the risk of CVD.

According to the statistics available from **CDC (Centre for Disease Control and Prevention)**, premature birth affects approximately 1 in 10 babies in United States.

Researchers analyzed existing data on 70182 women from the **Nurses' Health Study-2**: one of the largest ongoing studies into the risk factors for major chronic diseases in women. The study revealed that preterm delivery correlated with a 40 % higher risk of developing CVD compared with women who gave birth at term. The risk increased for women who had more than one preterm delivery. Women who delivered earlier than 32 weeks had double the risk of developing CVD.

According to the **American Heart Association (AHA),** women already have a risk of dying from CVD of 33 %. This number rises to 36 % for those who give birth 3-7 weeks before term and rises as 60 % for women who deliver 8 weeks or more prematurely.

Several factors contribute to this association:

o **Inflammation and oxidative stress:** Preterm delivery can cause stress on the maternal cardiovascular system, leading to increased inflammation and oxidative stress which are known risk factors for CVD.

o **Association with pre-eclampsia:**
Sometimes pregnancy is terminated prematurely for uncontrolled severe pre-eclampsia. Pre-eclampsia itself is linked to increased risk of CVD.

Link Between Preterm Delivery and Cardiovascular Risk Later in Life

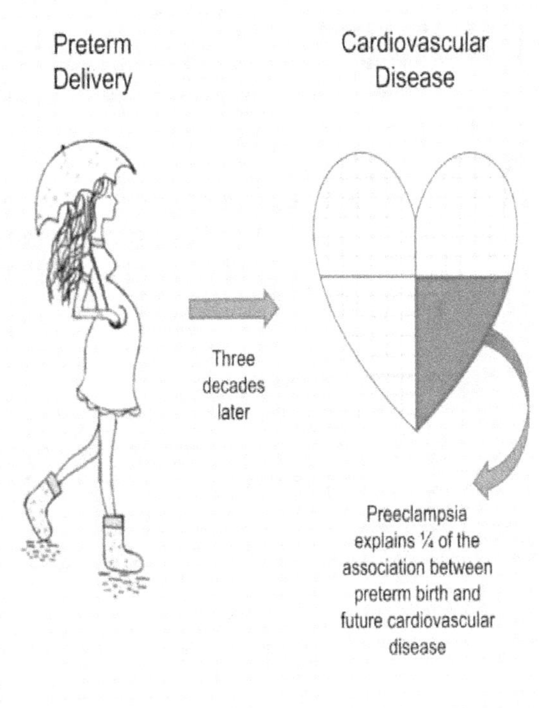

Link Between Multiple Pregnancy Losses and the Risk of CVD Later in Life

Research has shown that there might be a link between multiple pregnancy losses (Recurrent miscarriages and stillbirths) and the risk of CVD later in life for women. The potential mechanisms linking multiple pregnancy losses and CVD are not fully understood, but several factors do play a role.

- o **Chronic Stress:**
  Going through multiple pregnancy losses can lead to chronic stress which may contribute to inflammation and negatively affect cardiovascular health.

- o **Immune System Dysregulation:**
  Multiple pregnancy losses may trigger immune system, potentially leading to inflammation and other CVD risk factors.

- o **Shared Risk Factors:**
  Women who experience multiple pregnancy losses may have other underlying health conditions like hypertension, diabetes or risk factors that can also increase their CVD risk.

Link Between age at Menarche and the Risk of CVD Later in Life

Menarche, a first menstruation, is the milestone event of pubertal development in girls since it represents the onset of female reproductive capacity.

Menarche is a complex phenomenon that is influenced by genetic and environmental factors.

According to the recent review, the age at menarche has remained stable between 12-16 years over the past few decades.

Age at menarche has been studied in relation to CVD risk later in life. Several research studies have explored this association. The exact mechanism behind this association is not fully understood, but it is believed that hormonal and metabolic changes during puberty may influence CVD health later in life.

In Korean population, menarche before 12 years (precocious menarche) has been linked to increased prevalence of obesity, insulin resistance and dyslipidemia in adulthood, culminating in higher CVD risk.

In a large population-based study in China, it has been found that those who had late menopause (after 15 years) had a higher risk of obesity, hypertension, diabetes and CVD risk compared with other women.

Link Between PCOS (polycystic ovarian syndrome) and Risk of CVD Later in Life.

Polycystic Ovarian Syndrome is a disease that affects the endocrine, metabolic and reproductive systems and manifest in the reproductive age group.

The global prevalence of PCOS is estimated between 4% and 20%. The World Health Organization **(WHO)** data suggests that approximately 116 million women are affected by PCOS globally.

Common Clinical Presentations of PCOS Include:

- **Irregular or infrequent menstrual cycles**
  Women with PCOS often experience irregular and infrequent menstrual cycles, which can lead to difficulty in predicting the ovulation resulting difficulty in conceiving and present in the clinics to seek advice for conception.

- **Weight Gain**
  Many women with PCOS find it difficult to lose weight, especially around abdomen.

- **Excessive hair growth**
  Increased levels of androgens in PCOS can lead to hirsutism (excessive hair growth on face, chest, back etc.)

- **Acne and oily skin**
  Elevated androgens can also contribute to the development of acne and oily skin.

Several Factors Contribute PCOS Association with CVD Later in Life:

Insulin Resistance:

Many women with PCOS have insulin resistance, a condition where the body cells do not respond effectively to insulin. Insulin resistance can lead to higher levels of insulin and glucose in the blood stream, increasing the risk of type 2 diabetes and metabolic syndrome. Both these conditions are risk factors for CVD.

Obesity:

PCOS is often linked with obesity, and excess weight can contribute to insulin resistance, inflammation and other factors that raise the risk of CVD.

Dyslipidemia:

PCOS can lead to changes in lipid profile, including elevated levels of LDL-C and triglycerides; and reduced levels of HDL-C. Imbalances in lipid levels are associated with an increased risk of CVD.

Inflammation:

PCOS is associated with chronic low-grade inflammation in the body. Inflammation plays a role in the development of atherosclerosis and increases the risk of CVD.

Androgen levels:

Elevated levels of androgen in PCOS can contribute to insulin resistance, dyslipidemia and inflammation, all of which are risk factors for CVD.

Endothelial Dysfunction:

PCOS may lead to endothelial dysfunction. Endothelial dysfunction is early marker of cardiovascular disease.

Link between autoimmune diseases and CVD later in life

Autoimmune diseases are conditions in which the body's immune system mistakenly attacks healthy cells, tissues and organs leading to inflammation and damage. There are numerous types of autoimmune diseases including rheumatoid arthritis, systemic lupus erythematosus (SLE), multiple sclerosis, psoriasis etc.

80 % of all individuals affected by autoimmune diseases tend to be women due to variation within the sex chromosomes (XX) and hormonal changes.

- o **Every 10 patients diagnosed with SLE, 9 are women.**

- o **Out of every 7 patients diagnosed of rheumatoid arthritis, 5 are women.**

- o **Systemic Sclerosis is 4 times more likely to occur in women.**

An International Research Team led by KU Leuven published the results of an epidemiological investigation into possible links between 19 of the most common autoimmune diseases and CVD. The results showed that patients with autoimmune disorder have a substantial higher risk **(between 1.4 to 3.6 times)** of developing CVD than people without autoimmune disorder.

Factors contributing the risks for developing CVD.

- The connection between autoimmune disease and the risk of CVD is postmenopausal women is primarily due to chronic inflammation. When the immune system remains in a state of constant activation, it releases inflammatory molecules that can damage blood vessels and promote the development of atherosclerosis.

- Atherosclerosis can lead to the formation of plaques within the arterial walls, which restrict blood flow to the heart causing heart attack or brain causing stroke; it can be life-threatening.

- Postmenopausal women are already at an increased risk of CVD due to hormonal changes associated with menopause. When risk due to autoimmune disease is added to the mix, the risk is further amplified.

CHAPTER V: WORK-UP FOR ASSESSING THE RISK FACTORS FOR CVD AT MENOPAUSE CLINIC

"The journey through menopause brings new challenges to heart health, but with knowledge and care, women can rewrite their cardiovascular story."

The aim of establishing menopausal clinics is to screen and diagnose specific menopause-related problems and to assess the general condition of a woman by history, clinical examination and basic laboratory tests and plan for individualized management strategies.

The menopause transition or perimenopause is the **"Window of Opportunity"** to screen and to treat women for non-communicable diseases.

The concept of menopausal health is about women getting and staying healthy throughout life and should celebrate postmenopausal life with strength, energy and certain goals.

The Centre for Disease Control and Prevention urges all women to make healthy living a priority.

At menopause clinic primary healthcare provider is a gynecologist who takes detailed history, does physical examination including pelvic and breast examination, investigates her, identifies risk factors and formulate a plan for individualized counseling and treatment. The approach is basically multi-speciality oriented.

Here we will only discuss the points which are in relation with assessing **the potential risk factors in causation of cardiovascular events in future in postmenopausal women.**

(A)History Taking for Finding out Risk Factor for CVD:

Screening postmenopausal women for cardiovascular health risks in a Menopausal Clinic requires a comprehensive approach involving detailed history taking, clinical examination, blood investigations, and imaging modalities. Here is how to approach each component.

Personal Medical History:

o   Hypertension
o   Dyslipidemia
o   Diabetes
o   Previous cardiovascular events if any
o   Chronic kidney disease
o   Autoimmune diseases like rheumatoid arthritis, SLE etc.
o   Sleep apnea

Reproductive History:

o   Age at menarche
o   Polycystic Ovarian Syndrome (PCOS)
o   Pregnancy complications if any
    ▪   Gestational hypertension/Pre-eclampsia
    ▪   Gestational diabetes
    ▪   Preterm delivery
    ▪   Multiple pregnancy losses

Menopausal History:

o   Age at menopause
o   Symptoms, if any
o   Hormone Replacement Therapy (HRT) usage, including its duration and type

Lifestyle Factors:

o   Dietary habits
o   Physical activity level
o   Smoking
o   Alcohol consumption
o   Stress levels and sleep pattern

Present Medication History:

o   Use of blood pressure medications
o   Use of cholesterol lowering medications
o   Medications for diabetes
o   Chronic use of any other medications that may influence cardiovascular risk (e.g. NSAIDs, oral contraceptive etc.)

Psychological Factors:

o   Chronic stress
o   Anxiety and depression

Family medical history:

o   Cardiovascular diseases (e.g. heart attack, stroke) in parents, siblings and close relatives.
o   Cardiovascular events earlier in life in family members.

(B)Physical Examination:

Physical examination should focus on identifying signs and markers that could indicate increased risk of cardiovascular events. It should be comprehensive and tailored to the individual's medical history and risk factors. Here are some points to be included in physical examination.

Blood Pressure Measurement:

Obtain accurate blood pressure readings to assess for hypertension, a major risk factor for cardiovascular disease. (Normal Blood Pressure: 120/80 mm of Hg.)

Body Mass Index (BMI) Calculation:

Calculate BMI: weight in kg/ (height in meter) 2 to evaluate weight status and potential obesity-related risks. (Normal BMI: 18.5 – 24.9 kg/m2).

Waist Circumference:

Measure waist circumference and waist-to-hip ratio to assess central adiposity (visceral adiposity), which is associated with increased CVD risk. (Normal waist circumference: <80 cms and waist-to-hip ratio < 0.85 as per WHO criteria.)

Palpation of Peripheral Pulses:

Check peripheral pulses (e.g. radial, femoral, pedal) to assess for peripheral arterial disease.

Auscultation of Heart Sounds:

Listen for abnormal heart sounds if any (murmur, extra heart sounds) that may indicate underlying heart conditions.

Assessment of Jugular Venous Pressure (JVP):

Examine JVP to assess for signs of heart failure or fluid overload.

Assessment of Thyroid Gland:

Palpate thyroid gland for any abnormality that could contribute to cardiovascular risk.

Examination of Lower Extremities:

Look for signs for edema, varicose veins and skin changes that might indicate circulatory issues.

Skin Examination:

Look for xanthomas (cholesterol deposits) and skin manifestations of lipid disorders.

Respiratory Examination:

Assess for signs of lung congestion or respiratory issues that could affect cardiovascular health.

Fundoscopic Examination by the Ophthalmologist:

Evaluate the retina for signs of hypertensive retinopathy or other vascular changes.

Neurological Examination:

Evaluate neurological status, including reflexes and sensations, which can provide insides into overall vascular health.

(C)Investigations:

In the cardiovascular risk assessment for postmenopausal women, the choice of investigations may vary based on the individual's risk factors and clinical presentation. Choice of investigations should be tailored to each individual's risk factors, symptoms and medical history. Here are some investigations that may be advised.

Blood Tests:

Lipid Profile:

Normal values:

- o   Total Cholesterol: < 200 mg/dl
- o   Triglycerides: < 150 mg/dl
- o   LDL-C: < 100 mg/dl
- o   HDL-C: > 40 mg/dl

Fasting Blood Sugar:

Normal values: < 100 mg/dl

HbA1C:

Monitors long-term glucose control: Normal values: Between 4 – 5.6 %. Levels between 5.7 and 6.4 suggest that you are prediabetes and a higher chance of getting diabetes.

High-Sensitive C - reactive protein (hs-CRP):

Measures inflammation: Normal value: less than 0.3 mg/dl. Minor elevation (0.3-1 mg/dl) can be seen in obesity, diabetes, sedentary lifestyle, cigarette smoking, pregnancy and genetic polymorphism.

Homocysteine Levels:

Evaluate vascular health: Normal value: Most lab reports normal ranges of homocysteine as about 4 – 15 microml/L.

Liver Function Tests:

To monitor lipid metabolism and rule out fatty liver disease, which is linked to cardiovascular health.

Thyroid Function Tests:

Detects deranged functions in relation to thyroid gland as both hyperthyroidism and hypothyroidism can affect cardiovascular health.

Renal Function Tests (RFT):

Detects deranged functions in relation to kidney. Chronic kidney disease is a risk factor for cardiovascular disease.

Electrolytes:

To assess conditions like hyperkalemia or hyponatremia that can affect heart health.

Complete Blood Count (CBC): Detects anemia and other blood related issues.

Imaging Modalities:

Following investigations are not mandatory and should be individualized and advised judiciously by cardiologist depending upon the risk factors and the presenting symptoms.

- o **Electrocardiogram (ECG):**
  A baseline ECG can detect arrhythmias, myocardial ischemia or other cardiac abnormalities.

- o **Echocardiogram:**
  Non-invasive evaluation of heart structure and function. It is especially useful if there are symptoms suggestive of heart disease, such as breathlessness or chest pain.

- o **Stress Test:**
  If the patient presents with exertional symptoms, a stress test (e.g. treadmill exercise ECG, stress echocardiography) may be necessary to assess for ischemic heart disease.

- o **Coronary Artery Calcium (CAC) Score (CT scan):**
  To quantify the extent of calcified plaques in coronary arteries, helping to stratify cardiovascular risk.

- o **Carotid Ultrasound:**
  This imaging can assess carotid intima-media thickness and the presence of atherosclerotic plaques, serving as surrogate marker for cardiovascular risk.

- o **DEXA Scan:**
  Though primarily for bone density assessment, it provides insights into body composition, including visceral fat, which is linked to cardiovascular risk.

Cardiovascular Risk Assessment Models for Detection of Long-Term Risk of CVD

Cardiovascular risk assessment models are tools designed to estimate an individual's long-term risk of developing cardiovascular disease (CVD). They incorporate various factors like age, sex, cholesterol levels, blood pressure, smoking status, and more. Here are some of the popular online and offline models used for assessing CVD risk.

Online Models:

1. Framingham Risk Score (FRS):

One of the most widely used models, it calculates 10-year cardiovascular risk based on factors like age, gender, cholesterol levels, blood pressure, diabetes and smoking status.

Link: Framingham Risk Score Calculator

2. QRISK3:

A UK based model that estimates the 10-year risk of developing CVD. It includes a broader range of risk factors, including ethnicity, chronic kidney disease and family history.

Link: QRISK3 Calculator

3. American College of Cardiology/American Heart Association (ACC/AHA) ASCVD Risk Calculator:

Estimates 10-year and lifetime risk for atherosclerotic cardiovascular disease using factors like cholesterol levels, blood pressure and lifestyle.

Link: ASCVD Risk Estimator

4. Heart Age Calculator

Provides an estimate of the patient's 'heart age' based on traditional risk factors.

By systematically screening postmenopausal women using these methods, clinicians in a Menopause Clinic can identify women at increased cardiovascular risk and implement early preventive measures, including lifestyle modifications, medical therapy and regular monitoring.

CHAPTER VI: LIFESTYLE MODIFICATIONS TO REDUCE THE CHANCES OF CARDIOVASCULAR DISEASE

"Heart health in postmenopausal women is a lifelong commitment, starting with understanding the changes and making mindful choices every day."

By adopting a healthy lifestyle, you can help keep your blood pressure, cholesterol, blood sugars and body weight within normal limits; and lower your risk of heart attacks.

Although some factors like age and genetics are beyond our control, 80 % of the risk of cardiovascular disease can be prevented by healthy eating and regular physical activities.

People are relying on vitamins and minerals rather than diet, exercise and healthy lifestyle and that's probably not good.

Here are some lifestyle changes that postmenopausal women can adopt to help reduce the risk of cardiovascular disease.

(A)Heart-friendly Diet:

A heart-friendly diet for postmenopausal women should focus on maintaining a healthy weight, managing cholesterol levels, thereby promoting overall health. Here are some of the dietary guidelines.

- **Increase Fiber Intake**
  Increase whole grains, fruits, green vegetables, legumes and nuts in your diet. High fiber foods help lower cholesterol level and improve heart health.

- **Choose Healthy Fats**
  Opt for sources of unsaturated fats like olive oil, avocados and nuts. Limit saturated and trans fats found in fried foods and processed snacks.

- **Lean Proteins**
  Choose lean protein sources like fish, skinless poultry, beans and lentils. Fish rich in omega-3 fatty acids (such as salmon) can be particularly beneficial for heart.

- **Reduce Sodium**
  Limit your sodium intake to help manage blood pressure. Avoid processed foods, canned soups and excess salts in cooking.

- **Increase Omega-3 fatty acids**
  Consume sources of omega-3 fatty acids, such as fatty fish, flaxseeds, chia seeds and walnuts to reduce inflammation and support heart health.

- **Limit added sugars**
  Minimize sugary foods and beverages as they can contribute to weight gain and increase the risk of heart disease.

- **Control Portion Sizes**
  Be mindful of portion sizes to avoid overeating and manage weight effectively.

- **Choose low-fat dairy**
  Opt for low fat or non-fat dairy products to reduce saturated fat intake.

- **Colorful Variety**
  Consume a colorful array of fruits and vegetables to get a wide range of antioxidants, vitamins and minerals.

- **Stay hydrated**
  Drink plenty of water throughout the day to support overall health.

Fiber-rich foods help lower cholesterol levels and improve heart health. Here are some excellent sources of dietary fiber.

Legumes:
- Lentils
- Chickpeas
- Black beans
- Kidney beans
- Pinto beans

Whole Grains:
- Oats
- Quinoa
- Brown rice
- Whole wheat pasta
- Barley

Fruits
- Apples (with skin)
- Pears (with skin)
- Berries (raspberries, blackberries, strawberries)

- Oranges
- Bananas

Vegetables
- Broccoli
- Brussels sprouts
- Carrots
- Spinach
- Kale

Nuts and Seeds:
- Almonds
- Chia seeds
- Flaxseeds
- Sunflower seeds
- Pistachios

Whole Grain Cereals:
- Bran cereals (like bran flakes)
- Whole grain oat cereals

Whole Grain Bread:
- Look for bread labeled as "whole grain or whole wheat"

Popcorn:
- Air-popped popcorn is a whole grain snack high in fiber. (with no butter)

Dry Fruits:
- Prunes
- Raisins
- Dried apricots (consume in moderation due to natural sugars)

Sweet Potatoes:
An excellent source of fiber and vitamins.

Inclusion of healthy sources of fats (unsaturated fats) in diet is important for overall health and wellbeing. Here are some examples of healthy fatty foods that you can incorporate in your meals.

Avocado

Avocados are rich in monounsaturated fats, which are heart-friendly fats that can help improve cholesterol levels.

Olive oil

Olive oil is a staple of Mediterranean diet and is high in monounsaturated fats. It is used for cooking and drizzling over salads.

Nuts

Almonds, walnuts, pistachios and other nuts are sources of healthy fats, fiber and various nutrients.

Seeds

Chia seeds, flaxseeds and pumpkin seeds are rich in omega-3 fatty acids and provide a boost of healthy fats, fiber and nutrients.

Fatty fish

Salmon, mackerel, sardines and trout are excellent sources of omega-3 fatty acids, which have been shown to support heart and brain health.

Coconut

Coconut oil and coconut products can be used in cooking and baking. Coconut contains medium-chain triglycerides that are metabolized differently by the body.

Seaweed
Seaweed and algae-based products like spirulina are sources of healthy fats, minerals and antioxidants.

Dark chocolates
Dark chocolate with high cocoa content (70 % or higher) contains healthy fats and antioxidants. Enjoy in moderation.

Chia pudding
Chia seeds soaked in liquid (such as almond milk) create a pudding that's high in healthy fats and fiber.

Olives
Olives are rich in monounsaturated fats and can be added to salads, sandwiches and Mediterranean dishes.

Eating more saturated or unhealthy fats can raise your cholesterol levels and increase your risk of heart disease. Hence there should be restricted use of saturated fats in diet. Average woman should not eat more than 20 gms of saturated fats per day. Here are some examples of unhealthy or saturated fats containing food:

- Butter, ghee, cheese
- Processed foods like biscuits, cakes, chips etc.
- Fatty cuts of meat
- Pastries such as pies, quiches, sausage rolls
- Cream, crème fraiche, sour cream
- Ice cream, milkshakes

How to avoid trans fats?

Trans fats are the worst type of fats as they raise LDL-C and lowers HDL-C in our body. Trans fats have been linked to high blood pressure, diabetes, dyslipidemia, obesity and ultimately to heart disease.

- Avoid using "Vanaspati" ghee for any type of cooking.
- When deep frying foods like Puri, Pakoda, Samosa etc., do not heat the oil for longer time.
- Avoid leaving the food in the oil for a longer period.
- **Do not reheat the oil or reuse the same oil for frying.** The oil which has been once used for frying, can be used for preparation of vegetables, dal etc.

Fruits Preferred to Reduce Chances of Diabetes/Cardiovascular Disease

The glycemic index (GI) is a numerical scale that measures how quickly carbohydrate-containing foods raise blood sugar levels after consumption. The scale ranges from 0 to 100, with higher values indicating foods that cause a rapid spike in blood sugar. Foods with a low GI (55 or less) result in slower digestion and absorption, causing a slow rise in blood sugar. Conversely, foods with high GI (70 or more) lead to a quick and sharp rise in blood sugar levels.

Classification of Fruits by Glycemic Index

Low Glycemic Index Fruits (55 or less):

These fruits are absorbed more slowly, causing a gradual increase in blood sugar, which is beneficial for people looking to reduce the risk of diabetes and cardiovascular disease.

1. Cherries (GI: 20)

2. Grapefruit (GI: 25)

3. Apples (GI: 36)

4. Pears (GI: 38)

5. Oranges (GI: 40)

6. Strawberries (GI: 41)

7. Peaches (GI: 42)

8. Grapes (GI: 43)

9. Kiwi (GI: 52)

10. Blueberries (GI: 53)

Medium-Glycemic Index Fruits (56 – 69):

These fruits have moderate effect on blood sugar levels.

1. Pineapple (GI: 59)

2. Papaya (GI: 60)

3. Mango (GI: 56)

High Glycemic Index Fruits (70 or more):

1. Watermelon (GI: 76)

2. Ripe Bananas (GI: 70)

Fruits Preferred to Reduce Chances of Diabetes/Cardiovascular Disease

To reduce the risk of diabetes and cardiovascular diseases, it is advisable to include low-GI fruits in the diet. These fruits help maintain stable blood sugar levels and can contribute to overall heart health. Here are some fruits that are preferable:

Apples: Rich in fiber, vitamins and antioxidants, apples help regulate blood sugar.

Berries: (Strawberries, Blueberries etc.): High in fiber and antioxidants, they are excellent for heart health and blood sugar control.

Pears: High in fiber, pears aid in blood sugar regulation.

Oranges and Grapefruit: Contain fiber and vitamin C, contributing to heart health.

Cherries: Low GI and packed with antioxidants, cherries are good for reducing inflammation and maintaining blood sugar levels.

General Tips:

- Opt for whole fruits rather than fruit juices, as whole fruits contain fiber, which slows sugar absorption.

- Pair fruits with a protein or healthy fat source (e.g. nuts or yogurt) to further reduce their glycemic impact.

By focusing on low-GI fruits and maintaining a balanced diet, one can better manage blood sugar levels and reduce the risk of diabetes and cardiovascular disease.

(B)Heart-friendly Physical Activities for Prevention of Cardiovascular Events:

Engaging in regular physical activity is crucial for maintaining heart health. Here are some heart-friendly exercises. Healthcare provider may help you determine the appropriate level of exercise and may provide personalized recommendations based on your personal health need.

- **Aerobic Exercises:**
  Aim for at least 150 minutes of moderate-intensity aerobic exercise or 75 minutes of vigorous aerobic exercise per week. Activities can include brisk walking, jogging, swimming, cycling and dancing.

- **Walking:**
  Walking is a low impact exercise that can be easily incorporated into your daily routine. It helps improve cardiovascular fitness and supports weight management. **Walking is a wonderful drug. Walking for an average of 30 minutes daily or more can lower the risk of heart disease, stroke by 35% and type 2 diabetes by 40%.**

- **Swimming:**
  Swimming provides a full-body workout. It helps improve cardiovascular endurance, muscle strength and flexibility.

- **Cycling:**
  Cycling, whether outdoors or on a stationary bike, is a great way to improve heart health and leg strength. It's also a low-impact exercise.

- **Dancing:**
  Dance-based fitness classes or even dancing at home can be a fun and effective way to increase heart rate and improve cardiovascular fitness.

- **Strength Training:**
  Incorporate strength training exercises using light weights or resistance bands. Building muscle mass can help boost metabolism and improve overall health.

- **Yoga:**
  Yoga promotes flexibility, balance and relaxation.

- **Tai Chi:**
  This mind-body exercise combines slow, flowing movements with deep breathing. It helps improve balance, flexibility and relaxation.

- **Staying Active:**
  Engage in activities you enjoy, such as gardening, dancing around the house or playing with grandchildren. Every bit of movements adds up.

Why Aerobic exercises are considered as "Heart-Friendly"?

Aerobic exercises are considered heart-friendly because they provide a range of benefits that specifically target and improve cardiovascular health. It is important to start gradually and choose aerobic exercises that you enjoy and sustain. Do remember to warm up before exercising and cool down afterword to prevent injury. If you have any existing health conditions or concerns, it's a good idea to consult with a healthcare provider before beginning a new exercise. Here's why aerobic exercises are beneficial for your heart.

- **Strengthens the heart:**
  During aerobic activities, heart pumps more blood to supply oxygen and nutrients to the muscles and organs. Over the time, this strengthens the heart muscle, making it more efficient at pumping blood and improving overall cardiac function.

- **Improve Circulation:**
  Aerobic exercises help dilate blood vessels, which enhances blood flow through the body. This helps reduce the strain on blood vessels and lowers blood pressure, reducing risk of heart diseases.

- **Increase in Cardiac Output:**
  Cardiac output is the amount of blood, heart pumps per minute. Aerobic exercises increase cardiac output by making the heart beat more efficiently and effectively, which can result in better circulation.

- **Lower Cholesterol Levels:**
  Regular exercise can help raise levels of HDL-C, often referred to as good cholesterol and lower levels of LDL-C, known as bad cholesterol. This contributes to a healthier lipid profile which is needed to keep cardiovascular system healthier.

- **Weight Management:**
  Engaging in aerobic activities burns calories and helps with weight management. Maintaining a healthy weight reduces the risk of conditions like high blood pressure, diabetes and heart disease.

- **Enhance Oxygen Utilization:**
  Aerobic exercises improve your body's ability to use oxygen efficiently.

- **Reduce Inflammation:**
  Regular aerobic exercise can help reduce chronic inflammation, a factor that plays a role in the development of cardiovascular disease.

- **Stress Reduction:**
  Aerobic activities stimulate the release of endorphins, which are natural mood lifters. Reduced stress contributes to better heart health.

- **Better Blood Sugar Control:**
  Aerobic exercise improves insulin sensitivity, helping to regulate blood sugar levels. This particularly important for preventing or managing diabetes, which can impact heart health.

- **Long-term Heart Health:**
  Engaging in consistent aerobic activities over time contributes in maintaining heart health and reducing the risk of cardiovascular events such as heart attacks and strokes.

(C)Avoid Smoking

Smoking is a major risk factor for developing cardiovascular diseases (CVD), including coronary heart disease, stroke and peripheral artery disease. Here is how smoking affects cardiovascular health:

Increase Heart Rate and Blood Pressure:

Nicotine, a key component in cigarette, causes temporary increase in heart rate and blood pressure. This leads to heart working harder than normal, contributing to heart strain.

Damage Blood Vessels:

Smoking causes damage to the lining of the arteries, leading to the build-up of fatty deposits known as atherosclerosis. This narrows the arteries, restricting blood flow to the heart and other vital organs, potentially leading to heart attacks or stroke.

Reduces Oxygen Supply:

The carbon monoxide present in cigarette smoke binds with hemoglobin in blood, reducing its capacity to carry oxygen. This means heart has to pump harder to supply enough oxygen throughout the body.

Increases Blood Clotting:

Smoking increases the stickiness of platelets, the components of blood responsible for clotting. This heightens the risk of forming clots, which can obstruct blood flow and result in heart attacks or strokes.

Elevate Cholesterol Levels:

Smoking lowers the level of HDL, known as good cholesterol. This imbalance contributes to plaque build-up in arteries.

How to Quit Smoking?

Quitting smoking is a challenging but crucial step in reducing cardiovascular risk. Here are some strategies that can help:

Set a Quit Date:

Choose a specific date to quit smoking. Prepare for it by removing all smoking-related items like cigarettes, lighters and ashtrays from your surroundings.

Understand Your Triggers:

Identify situations, emotions or activities that make you crave a cigarette. Once you know your triggers, you can develop strategies to manage them, such as chewing gum or engaging in physical activities.

Use Nicotine Replacement Therapy (NRT):

Options like nicotine gum, patches, inhalers or nasal sprays help reduce withdrawal symptoms and cravings by providing small doses of nicotine without the harmful chemicals in cigarettes.

Medications:

Certain prescription medications, such as varenicline (Chantix) and bupropion (Zyban), can help reduce withdrawal symptoms and the pleasure associated with smoking.

Seek Support:

Join a support group, whether online or in person. Sharing experiences with others who are also trying to quit can provide emotional support and encouragement. Professional counseling and smoking cessation programs are also beneficial.

Stay Active:

Engage in regular physical activity to manage stress, reduce cravings and improve overall health. Exercise releases endorphins, which can improve mood and make it easier to cope with withdrawal symptoms.

Avoid Alcohol and Caffeine:

These substances can trigger cravings for a cigarette. Reducing or avoiding their consumption, especially in the early stages of quitting, can help maintain focus on your goal.

Relapse is a Part of Process:

If you slip up and have a cigarette, don't be discouraged. Use it as a learning experience, identify what led to the relapse, and again renew your commitment to quit.

By quitting smoking, you significantly reduce the risk of cardiovascular disease. Within a year of quitting, the risk of heart disease drops by about half, and after 15 years, it becomes almost equivalent to that of a non-smoker.

(D)Avoid Sedentary Lifestyle:

Sedentary lifestyle, characterized by prolonged sitting or inactivity with minimal physical movement, poses a significant risk to cardiovascular health. The link between sedentary behaviour and cardiovascular disease (CVD) arises due to multiple factors.

Reduced Blood Circulation:

Prolonged sitting or lack of movements leads to poor circulation. This can result in blood pooling in the legs and reduced blood flow to the heart, increasing the risk of blood clots and deep vein thrombosis.

Impact on Heart Health:

Physical inactivity can lead to higher blood pressure and increased cholesterol levels, primary risk factors for heart disease. Regular exercise helps maintain a healthy blood pressure and improve cholesterol levels, but a sedentary lifestyle negates these benefits.

Weight Gain and Obesity:

Inactivity often leads to weight gain, as fewer calories are burned throughout the day. Excess weight, particularly around the abdomen, is directly linked to increased cardiovascular risk. Obesity also promotes metabolic disorders like type 2 diabetes, which further exacerbates cardiovascular risks.

Negative Metabolic Changes:

A sedentary lifestyle contributes to insulin resistance, which can lead to increased blood sugar levels. Over the time, this can result in metabolic conditions like diabetes, further heightening the risk of cardiovascular disease.

Inflammation:

Physical inactivity may lead to chronic low-grade inflammation, which is known contributor to atherosclerosis. This condition is a significant factor in the development of heart attacks and strokes.

Stand, stretch or walk every 30 minutes if your profession requires prolonged sitting (e.g. IT engineers working with laptops hours together).

Maintaining an active lifestyle is key to promoting heart heath and preventing cardiovascular disease associated with sedentary behaviour.

(E)Avoid Unhealthy Sleep Pattern:

Sleep plays a crucial role in maintaining cardiovascular health. Both insufficient and excessive sleep are associated with an increased risk of cardiovascular diseases.

Here is how sleep affects heart health:

Blood Pressure Regulation:

During sleep, blood pressure dips by 10-20%, known as nocturnal dipping. This rest period allows the heart to recover and reduces the overall stress on cardiovascular system. Poor or inadequate sleep disturbs this natural dip, leading to consistently high blood pressure, a major risk factor for heart disease.

Impact on Heart Rate and Rhythm:

Proper sleep helps regulate heart rate and rhythm. Sleep deprivation can increase risk of arrhythmias, which can lead to complications like heart attacks and strokes.

Inflammatory Response:

Chronic sleep deprivation triggers an inflammatory response in the body. Elevated levels of inflammation markers, such as C-reactive protein, are associated with the development of atherosclerosis.

Glucose Metabolism and Insulin Sensitivity:

Inadequate sleep can lead to insulin resistance, where the body becomes less effective at processing glucose. This condition contributes to higher blood sugar levels, increasing the risk of developing type 2 diabetes and metabolic syndrome, both of which are linked to cardiovascular disease.

Stress Hormones:

Poor sleep quality or short sleep duration increases the production of stress hormones like cortisol. Elevated cortisol levels contribute to increased blood pressure and can accelerate plaque build-up in the arteries, heightening cardiovascular risks.

Obesity and Weight Gain:

Lack of sleep affects the hormones that regulate hunger, leading to an increase in appetite and cravings for high-calorie foods. This can result in weight gain and obesity, both of which are significant risk factors for heart disease.

Sleep Disorders and Cardiovascular Risk:

Conditions like obstructive sleep apnea (OSA) are directly linked to cardiovascular risks. OSA causes repeated interruptions in breathing during sleep, leading to drops in blood oxygen levels and sudden increases in blood pressure. Over time, these disruptions contribute to the development of hypertension, arrhythmias, heart failure and stroke.

Promoting Heart Health Through Quality Sleep:

Maintain a Regular Sleep Schedule:

Going to bed and waking up at the same time each day helps regulate the body's internal clock and improve sleep quality.

Create a Restful Environment:

A quiet, dark and cool bedroom environment promotes uninterrupted sleep.

Limit Stimulants:

Reduce the intake of caffeine and alcohol, especially before bedtime, as they can interfere with normal sleep pattern.

Manage Sleep Disorders:

If experiencing symptoms like snoring, gasping during sleep or excessive daytime fatigue, seek medical evaluation for potential sleep disorders like sleep apnea.

Adequate sleep (typically 7 – 9 hours for most adults) and good sleep quality are vital for cardiovascular health, helping to regulate blood pressure, reduce inflammation and maintain heart function.

(F) Avoid Stress

The link between stress and cardiovascular health is well established, as chronic stress can negatively impact heart health in several ways. Here is a close look at how stress influences the cardiovascular system:

- **Physiological Effects of Stress on the Heart**

  - **Increased Heart Rate and Blood Pressure:**
    During stress the body releases stress hormones such as adrenaline and cortisol. These hormones prepare the body for a "fight or flight" response, causing an increase in heart rate and blood pressure. Chronic stress leads to persistent elevation in blood pressure, a significant risk factor for heart disease and stroke.

  - **Constricted Blood Vessels:**
    Stress hormones cause blood vessels to constrict, reducing blood flow to the heart. This can lead to temporary chest pain (angina) and increase the risk of heart attacks in those with existing coronary artery disease.

  - **Inflammation:**
    Chronic stress can trigger inflammation in the body. Inflammation plays a key role in the development of atherosclerosis, where arteries become clogged with fatty deposits, increasing the risk of heart attacks and other cardiovascular events.

- **Behavioral Responses to Stress and Cardiovascular Risk**

  o **Unhealthy Coping Mechanisms:**
  People under stress often engage in unhealthy behaviors, such as smoking, excessive alcohol consumption, overeating (especially high-fat, high-sugar foods), and physical inactivity. These habits contribute to the development of cardiovascular risk factors like obesity, hypertension, and high cholesterol.

  o **Poor Sleep Quality:**
  Stress often leads to sleep disturbances, including insomnia. Poor sleep is linked to increased risk of heart disease, as it affects blood pressure regulation, glucose metabolism, and overall heart health.

  o **Reduced Physical Activity:**
  Stress can lead to a lack of motivation to exercise. Physical inactivity is a known risk factor for cardiovascular disease, including heart attacks, stroke and hypertension.

- **Direct Impact on the Cardiovascular System**

  o **Increased Risk of Arrhythmias:**
  Chronic stress can disturb the heart's electrical activity, leading to arrhythmias or irregular heartbeats. Severe stress, such as during a traumatic event, can even trigger a condition known as "stress cardiomyopathy" or "broken heart syndrome", where the heart temporarily weakens.

  o **Blood Clotting:**
  Stress affects blood clotting mechanisms, increasing the risk of thrombosis (formation of blood clots). This

can lead to blockages in the coronary arteries, raising the risk of heart attacks and other cardiovascular complications.

- **Chronic Stress and Long-term Cardiovascular Health**
Long-term exposure to stress, particularly type of stress such as workplace stress, social isolation and financial strain, has been linked to the build-up of plaques and atherosclerosis.

- **Managing Stress to Protect Cardiovascular Health**
    - **Regular Exercise:** Physical activity can help reduce stress hormones and improve heart health.

    - **Healthy Diet:** Eating a balanced diet rich in fruits, vegetables and whole grains can mitigate the effects of stress on the cardiovascular system.

    - **Relaxation Techniques:** Practices like mindfulness, yoga, meditation and deep breathing exercises can help manage stress and reduce its impact on heart health.

    - **Social Support:** Managing strong social connections and seeking support during stressful times can lower stress levels and promote cardiovascular health.

In summary stress can have both direct and indirect effects on cardiovascular health. Chronic stress, particularly when combined with unhealthy coping mechanisms, increases the risk of developing heart disease, high blood pressure, arrhythmias and other cardiovascular issues. Managing stress through lifestyle changes and relaxation techniques is crucial for maintaining a healthy hearth.

(G) Avoid Excessive Alcohol Consumption

The link between alcohol and cardiovascular health is complex. Here is a breakdown of link between alcohol and Cardiovascular Health.

- **Excessive Alcohol Consumption and Cardiovascular Risks**

  - **High Blood Pressure:**
    Heavy drinking can lead to an increase in blood pressure, a significant risk factor for cardiovascular diseases, including stroke and heart attack.

  - **Cardiomyopathy:**
    Excessive alcohol consumption can weaken the heart muscle, leading to a condition called alcoholic cardiomyopathy, which affects the heart's ability to pump blood efficiently.

  - **Arrhythmias:**
    Heavy alcohol use can result in irregular heartbeats, such as atrial fibrillation, increasing the risk of stroke and other complications.

  - **Weight Gain and Diabetes:**
    Alcohol is high in calories and can lead to weight gain, increasing the risk of obesity and type 2 diabetes, both of which are major risk factors for cardiovascular disease.

- **Moderate Alcohol Consumption and Cardiovascular Health**

  o **Potential Benefits:**
    Some studies suggest that moderate alcohol consumption (up to one drink per day for women and up to two for men) may be associated with a reduced risk of certain cardiovascular conditions, particularly coronary artery disease (CHD). The possible benefits include:

    ✓ **Increased HDL Cholesterol:**
      Moderate alcohol intake has been linked to higher levels HDL cholesterol, which may help reduce the risk of heart disease.

    ✓ **Antioxidant Properties:**
      Certain alcoholic beverages, such as red wine, contain polyphenols like resveratrol, which have antioxidant properties that might benefit heart health by protecting the lining of blood vessels.

    ✓ **Reduced Blood Clot Formation:**
      Alcohol may have an anticoagulant effect, reducing the formation of blood clots that can lead to heart attacks and strokes.

- **No Universal Recommendation**
  While moderate consumption might offer some cardiovascular benefits, the potential risks often overweigh these benefits, especially for individuals with certain health conditions or a family history of alcohol addiction. Therefore, healthcare professionals typically recommend that individuals consider their overall health, risk factors and family history before

incorporating alcohol into their lifestyle for cardiovascular benefits.

In summary, the relationship between alcohol and cardiovascular health is dose-dependent, with moderate consumption potentially offering some protective effects, while excessive consumption poses significant risk to cardiovascular health.

(H)Monitor Health Parameters

- **Cheque Blood Pressure:**
  Regularly monitor blood pressure levels and manage them through diet, exercise and medications if needed as per the advice of healthcare professionals.

- **Monitor Cholesterol Levels:**
  Get regular blood tests to monitor cholesterol and triglyceride levels.

- **Keep Blood Sugar in Check:**
  Monitor blood sugar levels, especially if there is a risk of diabetes.

(I)Maintain a Healthy Weight

- **Calculate your BMI:**
  Aim to maintain a body mass index (BMI) within the normal range (18.5 – 24.9).

- **Adopt portion Control:**
  Be mindful of portion sizes to avoid overeating.

- **Focus on Gradual Weight Loss:**
  If overweight, aim for a slow and steady weight loss.

(J)Stay Hydrated

- **Drink Water:**
  Aim for at least 7 – 8 glasses of water per day to maintain overall bodily functions, including heart health

- **Limit Sugary Drinks:**
  Avoid excessive consumption of sugary beverages that can contribute to weight gain and diabetes.

Implementing these lifestyle modifications and following doctor's advice can significantly reduce the risk of developing cardiovascular diseases and promote overall heart health.

CHAPTER VII: PHARMACOLOGICAL INTERVENTIONS

"Menopause is not the end

but the beginning of new heart health journey

that requires awareness action and self-care"

Pharmacological interventions play a crucial role in reducing cardiovascular health risks, especially for those who cannot achieve optimum results through lifestyle changes alone. These medications are prescribed based on individual health profiles and must be taken under the strict advice and supervision of healthcare providers.

(A)Common Pharmacological Intervention:

1. **Antihypertensives:** These are used to manage high blood pressure, a major risk factor for cardiovascular diseases. Common classes of antihypertensives include:

- ACE inhibitors (e.g. Lisinopril, Enalapril) and ARBs (e.g. Losartan, Valsartan) help relax blood vessels.
- Beta-blockers (e.g. Metoprolol, Atenolol) reduce heart rate and the heart's workload.
- Calcium channel blockers (e.g. Amlodipine, Diltiazem) relax and widen blood vessels.
- Diuretics (e.g. Hydrochlorothiazide, Frusemide) help the body eliminate excess salt and water, reducing blood volume.

2. **Lipid-lowering Agents:** High cholesterol levels can contribute to buildup of plaque in arteries, increasing the risk of heart disease. Medications include:

- Statins (e.g. Atorvastatin, Rosuvastatin) lower LDL cholesterol and reduce the risk of heart attacks and strokes.
- Fibrates (e.g. Fenofibrate, Gemfibrozil) primarily lower triglycerides and increase HDL cholesterol.
- Cholesterol absorption inhibitors (e.g. Ezetimibe) decrease the absorption of dietary cholesterol in the intestines.

3. Antiplatelet Agents: These medications, like aspirin and Clopidogrel, prevent blood clots by inhibiting platelet aggregation. They are commonly recommended for individuals at high risk of cardiovascular events, such as those with a history of heart attacks or strokes.

4.Anticoagulants: Used to prevent blood clots in patients with conditions such as atrial fibrillation. Common examples include:

- Warfarin and newer oral anticoagulants (NOACs) like Apixaban and Rivaroxaban.

5.Blood Sugar Control: For individuals with diabetes, maintaining blood sugar within target ranges is crucial. Medications like Metformin and SGLT2 inhibitors not only manage blood sugar but also provide cardiovascular benefits.

It is essential to regularly monitor health parameters and follow the healthcare provider's advice for medication use, dosage adjustments, and potential side effects.

(B)Role of MHT (Menopause Hormone Therapy)

Key Points:

- Postmenopausal women have an increased risk of cardiovascular disease (CVD) due to the decline in estrogen levels, which plays a protective role in maintaining vascular health.

- Estrogen deficiency is associated with adverse changes in lipid profiles, endothelial dysfunction, and an increased risk of atherosclerosis, leading to a higher incidence of heart attacks and strokes.

- Estrogen have been shown to have major cardioprotective effects on women. This may be why it is less common to see women with CVD prior to menopause, after which estrogen levels drop sharply.

- This causal relationship is yet to be established clearly, as unfortunately MHT have not been successful in controlling this effect and may reflect a larger feedback loop in play to protect females from CVD in menopausal years.

- Initiation of MHT is a safe option for healthy asymptomatic women who are within 10 years of menopause or younger than 60 years of age and who do not have other contraindications to MHT.

- ***MHT is neither to be used for primary prevention (healthy postmenopausal women without CVD) nor for secondary prevention (postmenopausal women already suffering from CVD).***

- At any age, avoid MHT in women with high risk of CVD or with established CVD.

- MHT is effective in reducing vasomotor symptoms associated with perimenopause or menopause, promoting bone health and in many cases improving quality of life.

- A Cochrane review including 24 randomized controlled trials studying MHT administration for vasomotor symptoms demonstrated a reduction in weekly hot flashes by 75% and an 87% decrease in severity of hot flashes, demonstrating it **to be an effective therapy for this difficult-to-manage symptoms of menopause, which on its own is associated with increased risk of CVD.**

- MHT is cardioprotective, if started in perimenopause or early postmenopause for vasomotor symptoms in healthy women. It reduces the risk of type 2 diabetes and has positive effect on the lipid profile and metabolic syndrome.

- Randomized controlled data from a **Danish Osteoporosis Trials** have shown that MHT reduced the incidence of coronary heart disease by around 50% and reduced overall mortality if commenced within 10 years of menopause and below 60 years of age.

- **Early vs Late Intervention Trial with Estradiol (ELITE 2016)** reported that ET resulted in significantly lower risk of atherosclerosis progression when therapy initiated within 6 years of menopause. But this effect was not seen in the late postmenopausal women when therapy initiated 10 or more years after menopause.

- **The Kronos Early Estrogen Prevention Study (KEEPS)** evaluated the effectiveness of a combined estrogen / progestin in preventing progression of carotid intima-media thickness (CIMT) or coronary artery calcium (CAC) in women who are within 36 months of their final menstrual period.

- **The SMART (Selective Estrogen Menopause and Response to Therapy)** trials have gone a step further in evaluating effects of conjugated estrogens/bazedoxifene (Bazedoxifene 20 mg/CEE 0.45 mg) on postmenopausal women. At 12 months, this combination was associated with significant improvements in total cholesterol, LDL-C and HDL-C levels when compared with placebo. (Triglyceride levels, however were significantly increased).

CHAPTER VIII: CONCLUSION

"Empowering Women to Understand

the Link Between Menopause and Heart Disease Risk

During Postmenopausal Years"

The growing discussion about cardiovascular health in postmenopausal women is rooted in several key factors.

1. Increased Risk of CVD post-menopause:

Research has shown that after menopause, women experience a significant increase in the risk of cardiovascular diseases. This increase is partly due to decline in estrogen levels, which plays a protective role in maintaining heart health. Estrogen helps regulate blood pressure, cholesterol levels and arterial health. After menopause, the loss of this hormone increases vulnerability to heart conditions.

2. Changing Risk Factors:

With the transition into menopause, the risk factors such as weight gain, high blood pressure, insulin resistance and changes in cholesterol levels become more pronounced. These changes make it crucial to understand and address cardiovascular health during this stage of life.

3. Underestimation of Women's Heart Health:

Historically, heart disease was often considered a "man's disease", leading to a lack of awareness about its prevalence and impact on women. In recent years, the medical community has recognized the need to address this misconception, emphasizing the importance of cardiovascular health in women.

4. Early Detection and Prevention:

By focusing on cardiovascular health in postmenopausal women, healthcare professionals aim to promote early detection and prevention strategies. Lifestyle modifications, regular check-ups and management of risk factors can significantly reduce the risk of heart disease in this population.

5. Public Health Campaigns and Research:

Increased public health awareness campaigns and research into women's health have highlighted the gender-specific aspects of heart disease. This has spurred discussions around tailored interventions and care practices to address the unique cardiovascular health challenges faced by postmenopausal women.

6. Holistic Health Focus:

There is a growing emphasis on the holistic health of women, encompassing not just reproductive health but also chronic conditions that emerge with age, like cardiovascular diseases. This comprehensive approach encourages discussion around all aspects of postmenopausal health.

These factors together have brought cardiovascular health in postmenopausal women to the forefront of health discussions, underscoring the need for targeted education, research and healthcare practices.

CHAPTER IX: REFERENCES

1. *Saladin, Kenneth S. (2011). Human anatomy (3rd ed.). New York: McGraw-Hill. p. 520. ISBN 9780071222075.*

2. Jump up to:[a][b] *Saladin, Kenneth S. (2011). Human anatomy (3rd ed.). New York: McGraw-Hill. p. 540. ISBN 9780071222075.*

3. *How does the blood circulatory system work? – InformedHealth.org – NCBI Bookshelf. Institute for Quality and Efficiency in Health Care (IQWiG). 31 January 2019. Archived from the original on 29 January 2022.*

4. Jump up to:[a][b] *Sherwood, Lauralee (2011). Human Physiology: From Cells to Systems. Cengage Learning. pp. 401–. ISBN 978-1-133-10893-1. Archived from the original on 29 July 2020. Retrieved 27 June 2015.*

5. *Saladin, Kenneth S. (2011). Human anatomy (3rd ed.). New York: McGraw-Hill. p. 610. ISBN 9780071222075.*

6. *"The lymphatic system and cancer | Cancer Research UK". 29 October 2014. Archived from the original on 30 January 2022. Retrieved 30 January 2022.*

7. Cardiovascular+System at the U.S. National Library of Medicine Medical Subject Headings (MeSH)

8. *Pratt, Rebecca. "Cardiovascular System: Blood". Anatomy One. Amirsys, Inc. Archived from the original on 24 February 2017.*

9. Jump up to:[a][b][c][d] *Guyton, Arthur; Hall, John (2000). Guyton Textbook of Medical Physiology (10 ed.). Saunders. ISBN 978-0-7216-8677-6.*

10. Jump up to:[a][b] *Lawton, Cassie M. (2019). The Human Circulatory System. Cavendish Square Publishing. p. 6. ISBN 978-1-50-265720-6. Archived from the original on 28 January 2022. Retrieved 28 January 2022.*

11. *Gartner, Leslie P.; Hiatt, James L. (2010). Concise Histology E-Book. Elsevier Health Sciences. p. 166. ISBN 978-1-43-773579-6. Archived from the original on 28 January 2022. Retrieved 28 January 2022.*

12. *Alberts, B.; Johnson, A.; Lewis, J.; Raff, M.; Roberts, K.; Walters, P. (2002). Molecular Biology of the Cell (4th ed.). New York and London: Garland Science. ISBN 978-0-8153-3218-3. Archived from the original on 17 August 2006. Retrieved 30 August 2017.*

13. *Standring, Susan (2016). Gray's anatomy: the anatomical basis of clinical practice (Forty-first ed.). [Philadelphia]: Elsevier Limited. p. 1024. ISBN 9780702052309.*

14. *Iaizzo, Paul A (2015). Handbook of Cardiac Anatomy, Physiology, and Devices. Springer. p. 93. ISBN 978-3-31919464-6. Archived from the original on 11 October 2017. Retrieved 28 January 2022.*

15. *"A History of Women's Heart Health". American College of Cardiology. Archived from the original on 2020-12-03. Retrieved 2020-11-26.*

16. *Coulter, Stephanie A. (2011). "Epidemiology of Cardiovascular Disease in Women". Texas Heart Institute Journal. 38 (2): 145–147. ISSN 0730-2347. PMC 3066813. PMID 21494522.*

17. *Worrall-Carter L, Ski C, Scruth E, Campbell M, Page K (December 2011). "Systematic review of cardiovascular disease in women: assessing the risk". Nursing & Health Sciences. 13 (4): 529–535. doi:10.1111/j.1442-2018.2011.00645.x. PMID 22070582.*

18. *"How heart disease is different for women". Mayo Clinic. Retrieved 2022-09-12.*

19. *Filbey L, Khan MS, Van Spall HG (January 2022). "Protection by inclusion: Increasing enrollment of women in cardiovascular trials". American Heart Journal Plus: Cardiology Research and Practice. 13: 100091. doi:10.1016/j.ahjo.2022.100091. ISSN 2666-6022. PMC 10978184. S2CID 246453881.*

20. Jump up to:[a] [b] *Saeed A, Kampangkaew J, Nambi V (2017-10-01). "Prevention of Cardiovascular Disease in Women". Methodist DeBakey Cardiovascular Journal. 13 (4): 185–192. doi:10.14797/mdcj-13-4-185. PMC 5935277. PMID 29744010.*

21. *Dart A (2002-02-15). "Gender, sex hormones and autonomic nervous control of the cardiovascular system". Cardiovascular Research. 53 (3): 678–687. doi:10.1016/S0008-6363(01)00508-9. PMID 11861039. S2CID 19013807.*

22. *Robertson RM (May 2001). "Women and cardiovascular disease: the risks of misperception and the need for action". Circulation. 103 (19): 2318–2320. doi:10.1161/01.CIR.103.19.2318. PMID 11352875*

23. Jump up to:[a][b] *"Off-Campus Access: Login to e-Resources - McMaster Libraries". libraryssl.lib.mcmaster.ca. Retrieved 2022-04-06.*

24. Jump up to:[a][b][c] *Thomas JL, Braus PA (February 1998). "Coronary artery disease in women. A historical perspective". Archives of Internal Medicine. 158 (4): 333–337. doi:10.1001/archinte.158.4.333. PMID 9487230.*

25. *Mosca L, Hammond G, Mochari-Greenberger H, Towfighi A, Albert MA (March 2013). "Fifteen-year trends in awareness of heart disease in women: results of a 2012 American Heart Association national survey". Circulation. 127 (11): 1254–63, e1–29. doi:10.1161/CIR.0b013e318287cf2f. PMC 3684065. PMID 23429926.*

26. Jump up to:[a][b] *Cushman M, Shay CM, Howard VJ, Jiménez MC, Lewey J, McSweeney JC, et al. (February 2021). "Ten-Year Differences in Women's Awareness Related to Coronary Heart Disease: Results of the 2019 American Heart Association National Survey: A Special Report From the American Heart Association". Circulation. 143 (7): e239–e248. doi:10.1161/CIR.0000000000000907. PMC 11181805. PMID 32954796. S2CID 221828897.*

27. Jump up to:[a][b] *Christian AH, Rosamond W, White AR, Mosca L (2007-01-01). "Nine-year trends and racial and ethnic disparities in women's awareness of heart disease and stroke: an American Heart Association national study". Journal of Women's Health. 16 (1): 68–81. doi:10.1089/jwh.2006.M072. PMID 17274739.*

28. Crandall CJ, Mehta JM, Manson JE. Management of Menopausal Symptoms: A Review. JAMA. 2023 Feb 07;329(5):405-420. [PubMed]

29. Burkard T, Moser M, Rauch M, Jick SS, Meier CR. Utilization pattern of hormone therapy in UK general practice between 1996 and 2015: a descriptive study. Menopause. 2019 Jul;26(7):741-749. [PubMed]

30. Williams M, Richard-Davis G, Weickert A, Christensen L, Ward E, Schrager S. A review of African American women's experiences in menopause. Menopause. 2022 Nov 01;29(11):1331-1337. [PubMed]

31. Polo-Kantola P, Rantala MJ. Menopause, a curse or an opportunity? An evolutionary biological view. Acta Obstet Gynecol Scand. 2019 Jun;98(6):687-688. [PubMed]

32. Wang X, Wang L, Xiang W. Mechanisms of ovarian aging in women: a review. J Ovarian Res. 2023 Apr 06;16(1):67. [PMC free article] [PubMed]

33. Shifren JL. Genitourinary Syndrome of Menopause. Clin Obstet Gynecol. 2018 Sep;61(3):508-516. [PubMed]

34. Khandelwal S, Meeta M, Tanvir T. Menopause hormone therapy, migraines, and thromboembolism. Best Pract Res Clin Obstet Gynaecol. 2022 May;81:31-44. [PubMed]

35. Soares CN. Depression and Menopause: An Update on Current Knowledge and Clinical Management for this Critical Window. Med Clin North Am. 2019 Jul;103(4):651-667. [PubMed]

36. de Kruif M, Spijker AT, Molendijk ML. Depression during the perimenopause: A meta-analysis. J Affect Disord. 2016 Dec;206:174-180. [PubMed]

37. El Khoudary SR, Greendale G, Crawford SL, Avis NE, Brooks MM, Thurston RC, Karvonen-Gutierrez C, Waetjen LE, Matthews K. The menopause transition and women's health at midlife: a progress report from the Study of Women's Health Across the Nation (SWAN). Menopause. 2019 Oct;26(10):1213-1227. [PMC free article] [PubMed]

Previous Books Published in the Series, "Women's Health"

All books are available on Amazon.in as well as on Amazon.com.

Universal Link:

https://relinks.me/B0BW6ZVMXY

1.   Preconception Care Makes A Difference

"Preconception Care and Counselling is the window of opportunity to tackle all unhealthy maternal problems resulting in favorable environment for the growth of embryo/fetus."

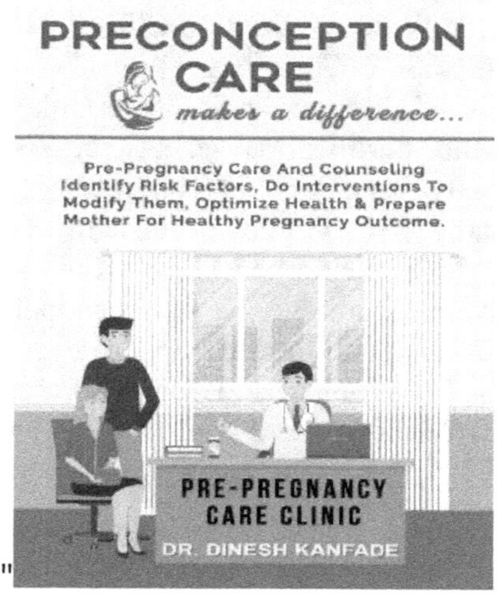

2. Understanding Menopause

"The biggest achievement of the last century is greater longevity that has resulted in an increased aged population worldwide. But the advantage of increased longevity is only when it is translated into healthy aging. Discover the secrets for understanding and managing menopause, thereby improving quality of life with this comprehensive updated guide."

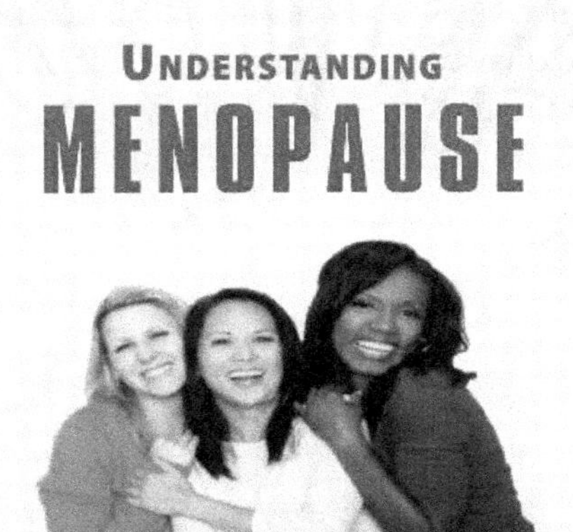

3. **Heart and Bone Health**

"We are living in aged population worldwide. It is obvious that women live significant part of their life after menopause. The ovaries of long years of dedicated service, have not the ability of retiring gracefully. But because of estrogen deficiency, ovaries become irritable and transmits this irritation to various organs of the body resulting in non-communicable diseases such as cardiovascular disease and osteoporosis. The advantage of increased longevity is only when it is translated into healthy aging. With a healthy lifestyle and understanding the pathophysiology of cardiovascular disease and osteoporosis in postmenopausal women, not only years will be added to increase the lifespan, but the extra years added will be of good quality. Discover the secretes of managing heart and bone health in postmenopausal women, thereby improving quality of life with this comprehensive guide."

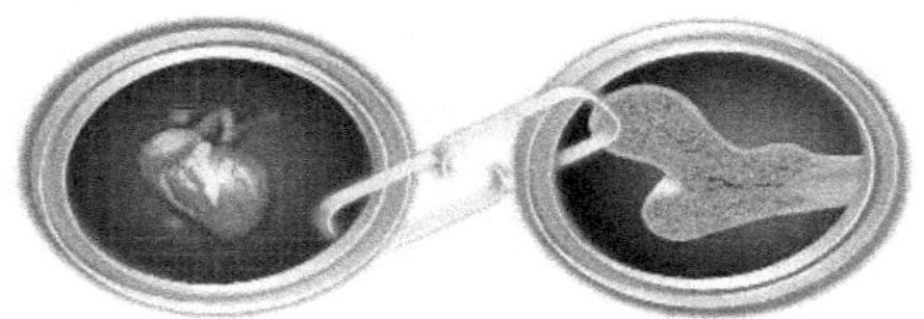

4. **Embracing Postmenopausal Intimacy**

"The postmenopausal phase, with its unique challenges and opportunities stands as a testament to the resilience of human intimacy. It is within this period of transformation that find an invitation to redefine and to rediscover physical closeness. Don't miss out on the transformative wisdom within these pages. Embrace the journey towards vibrant and fulfilling postmenopausal intimacy."

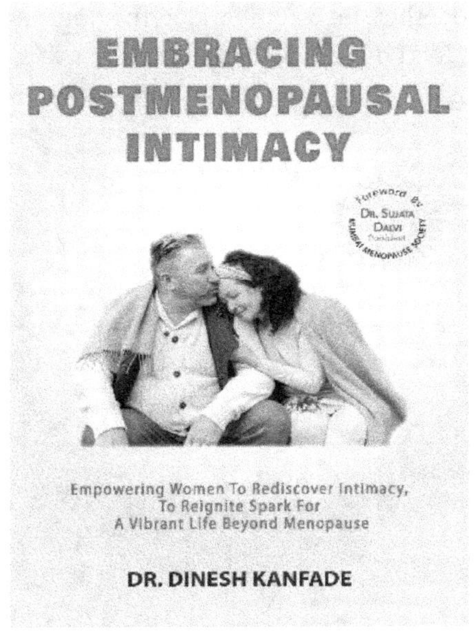

5. **Menstrual Health and Hygiene**

Unlock the secrets to optimal menstrual health and hygiene in this comprehensive guide.

From debunking myths to empowering insights, this book offers practical tips and evidence-based strategies for every stage of menstruation.

Whether you are seeking solutions for menstrual discomfort, navigating hygiene products or simply aiming for a healthier menstrual cycle, this book has covered everything you want in relation to menstruation.

Together, let us embark on this journey of enlightment, guided by the wisdom contained within these pages.

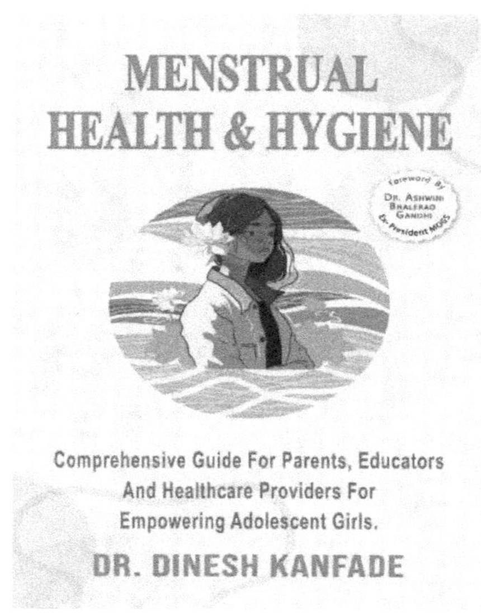

6. **The Silent Struggles: Understanding Women's Mental Health**

Mental health is often a quiet battle, and for women, it is a journey through the unique challenges at every stage of life.

The book is a comprehensive exploration of the emotional and psychological hurdles women face-from adolescence, through their reproductive years, to menopause.

The recurrence of heinous acts such as recent physical and sexual assault of junior doctor R. G. Kar Medical College Kolkata (August 2024), the infamous Nirbhaya case (2012) and many others suggest several concerning ground realities.

This book offers a profound understanding of how social, cultural and biological factors shape a woman's mental health.

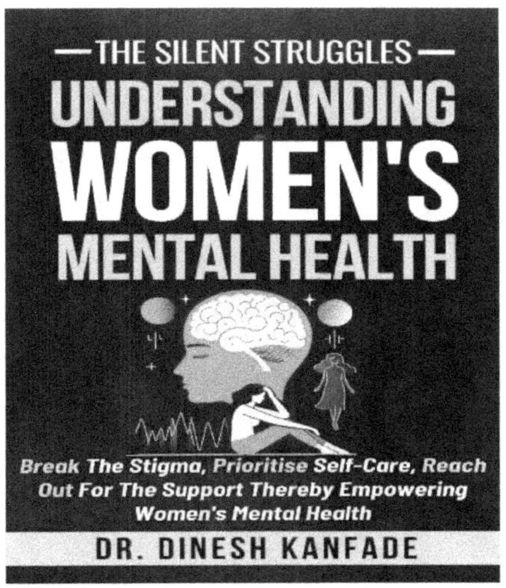

7. Nurturing Wellness: The Path to Breast Cancer Awareness

The breast has always been the symbol of womanhood and ultimate fertility. As a result, both disease and surgery of the breast evoke a fear of mutilation and loss of femininity.

Breast cancer remains a major health concern due to its high incidence worldwide and the significant impact it has on women's health.

This book contains vital information about the prevalence, prevention and tips for early detection of breast cancer for better survival rates.

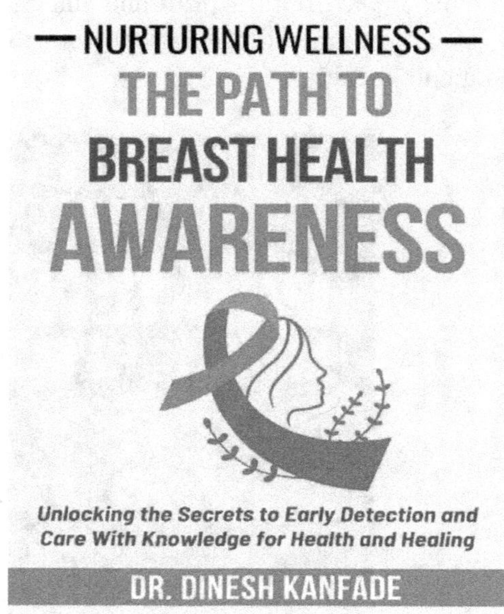